the ultimate
KETOGENIC
COOKBOOK

ELLA SANDERS

100 LOW-CARB, HIGH-FAT PALEO RECIPES for EASY WEIGHT LOSS and OPTIMUM HEALTH

CASTLE POINT BOOKS

NEW YORK

THE ULTIMATE KETOGENIC COOKBOOK
Copyright © 2018 by St. Martin's Press. All rights reserved.
Printed in the United States of America. For information,
address St. Martin's Press, 175 Fifth Avenue, New York, N.Y. 10010.

www.castlepointbooks.com
www.stmartins.com

The Castle Point Books trademark is owned by Castle Point Publications, LLC.
Castle Point books are published and distributed by St. Martin's Press.

ISBN 978-1-250-18380-4 (trade paperback)

Cover design by Katie Jennings Campbell
Interior design by Tara Long
Images provided by Allan Penn or used under license from Shutterstock.com
Recipes developed with the assistance of Shea Zukowski

Our books may be purchased in bulk for promotional, educational, or business use. Please contact your
local bookseller or the Macmillan Corporate and Premium Sales Department at 1-800-221-7945, extension 5442,
or by e-mail at MacmillanSpecialMarkets@macmillan.com.

First Edition: January 2018
10 9 8 7 6 5 4 3 2 1

contents

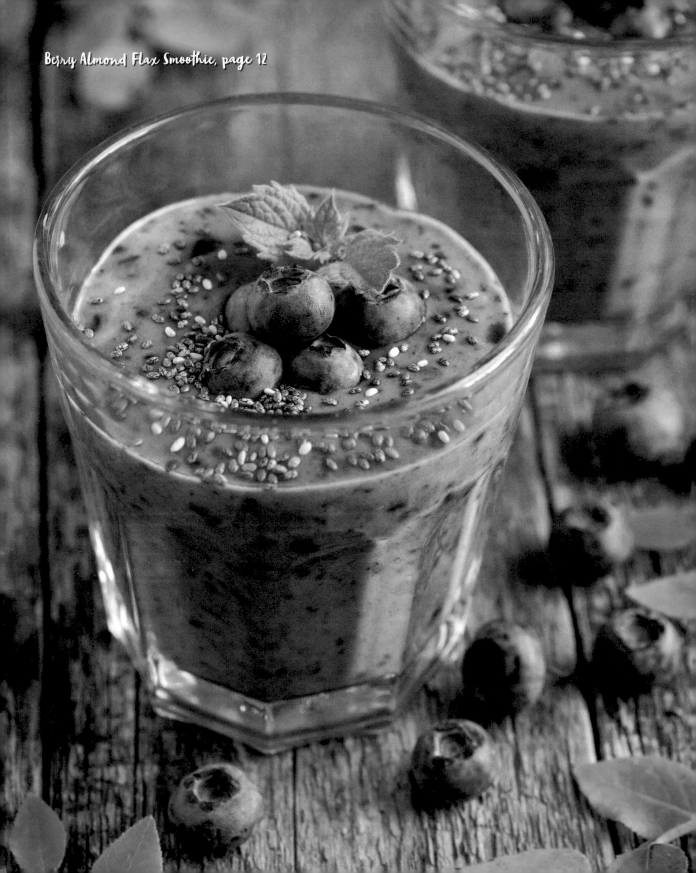

Berry Almond Flax Smoothie, page 12

chapter 1
KETO POWER AND FLAVOR

Keto Power and Flavor

If you're interested in a way to lose weight, feel great, improve your energy levels, and enjoy great-tasting food, then this book is for you! Here you'll find a delicious collection of easy-to-follow recipes that can help you do just that. Sound too good to be true? Give it a try for a few weeks and see how you feel. Most people experience dramatic results with this new way of eating.

So what exactly is a ketogenic diet?

A ketogenic diet is a very low-carb way of eating that helps the body use ketones instead of carbs for fuel. For years it was studied as a way to help people with epilepsy control their seizures. But along the way, experts also noticed a ketogenic diet promoted reliable weight loss as well.

Why does it work?

The term *ketosis* refers to a metabolic state in which your body uses ketones (taken from the fat you eat, as well as body fat) as its primary fuel source instead of glucose (from carbohydrates). When your body enters this fat-burning state, you naturally lower your blood sugar levels, which may be beneficial if you are at risk for developing diabetes. Low-carb diets have also been shown to help lower bad cholesterol levels and reduce high blood pressure, factors that may play a role in reducing the risk of heart disease.

Another benefit of a ketogenic weight loss plan: Because fats are more calorie dense, they help you feel full faster. And without the sudden insulin spikes that go along with eating lots of carbohydrates, you are far less likely to feel the usual hunger pangs we typically associate with trying to lose weight.

Do I need to talk with my doctor before starting a ketogenic diet?

It's always smart to talk with your doctor before starting any weight loss plan, especially if you are living with a chronic health condition like diabetes or heart disease. If you have seizures and are curious to try a ketogenic diet to see if they might be lessened, talk with your doctor to determine the carbohydrate goal that is best for you.

Sounds good so far. But what can I eat?

To help the body reach a state of ketosis, you'll want to focus on eating whole foods as much as possible, especially those low in carbohydrates and rich in healthy fats. That means you can enjoy olive oil, eggs, avocados, nuts, full-fat cheeses, and even the occasional butter splurge in your cooking! When it comes to vegetables, you can enjoy practically anything provided it isn't too starchy. Greens, mushrooms, broccoli, cabbage, cucumbers, tomatoes, zucchini, and yellow squash are all low-carb superstars that figure prominently into the recipes that follow.

In general, to achieve ketosis you should aim to get no more than 50 grams of carbohydrates a day and make sure that 70 percent of your calories are coming from fat. The recipes in this collection provide nutrition facts to help you keep track of macronutrients and calculate your overall daily intake. They also indicate the percentage of calories drawn from each macronutrient. You'll see that not every dish contains 70 percent of its calories from fat, but many contain more than that amount. Over the course of your day, strive for balance by eating a variety of low-carb foods. There are so many delicious choices!

What should I avoid?

To minimize the amount of carbohydrates you eat in a day, steer clear of the following:

- all grains and beans (including wheat flour, bread, pasta, and rice)
- all sweet and starchy vegetables (avoid all potatoes, peas, corn, and beets; limit onions and sweet peppers)
- all fruits (except berries)
- alcohol (including wine)
- added sugar (including honey, syrup, agave nectar; read labels carefully to avoid anything with sugar or high fructose corn syrup)

That may sound like a tall order, but take a look at the recipes in this collection. You'll see there is definitely a way to still enjoy many of your favorite comfort foods, such as pizza, burgers, and a variety of savory casseroles, as well as plenty of sweet treats and snacks to keep you satisfied between meals. After a short time, you're very likely to find this new way of eating so rewarding you wouldn't think of going back to your old recipes.

Are there any special foods on this plan?

For the most part, there's nothing out of the ordinary about the foods you'll eat on a ketogenic weight loss plan. In this collection of recipes, you may find it helpful to take note of the following:

AVOCADO. The easiest way to prepare this healthy-fat fruit is to slice it in half, turning it as you cut around the stone. Twist the two halves to separate them and then use a spoon to remove the stone and scoop the flesh from the skin.

BUTTER. Unless otherwise specified, use unsalted butter in your cooking; it is better to add a small amount of salt to a dish as you cook rather than rely on salty ingredients to enhance the flavor of your cooking. Over time, you may find that you add less salt to your food.

CHEESE. Because a ketogenic weight loss plan relies on the right ratio of fats in your diet, avoid reduced-fat cheeses unless the recipe specifies otherwise.

EGGS. Unless otherwise specified, use large eggs.

MEATS AND POULTRY. Some proponents of a ketogenic weight loss plan encourage using organic, grass-fed, or free-range animal products whenever possible; the choice is yours to make. However, unless otherwise specified, the recipe analysis assumes that ground beef is 85 percent lean and ground turkey is 93 percent lean.

NUTS. Toasted nuts make a statement in a dish (especially in a salad). To prepare them on the stovetop, simply cook the nuts in a dry skillet over medium-high heat for about 5 minutes, until fragrant. In the last minute or two, stir the nuts in the skillet. They can easily go from toasted to burnt in a matter of seconds.

OLIVE OIL. Use extra-virgin olive oil when you desire a more pronounced flavor in the finished dish (such as in a salad);

however, unless otherwise specified, the choice is up to you and your budget.

SWERVE. There are many granulated sugar replacements that claim they are zero-carbohydrate foods because the small amount they do contain is indigestible; in these recipes we call for a readily available brand called Swerve that looks and tastes very much like the real thing, but you can use any similar sugar-free product.

WHEY PROTEIN POWDER. Some recipes call for this product, which you'll find in the powdered energy-shakes aisle of your grocery or health food store. You can find it in a variety of flavors, but most of the desserts in this collection use a vanilla-flavored product.

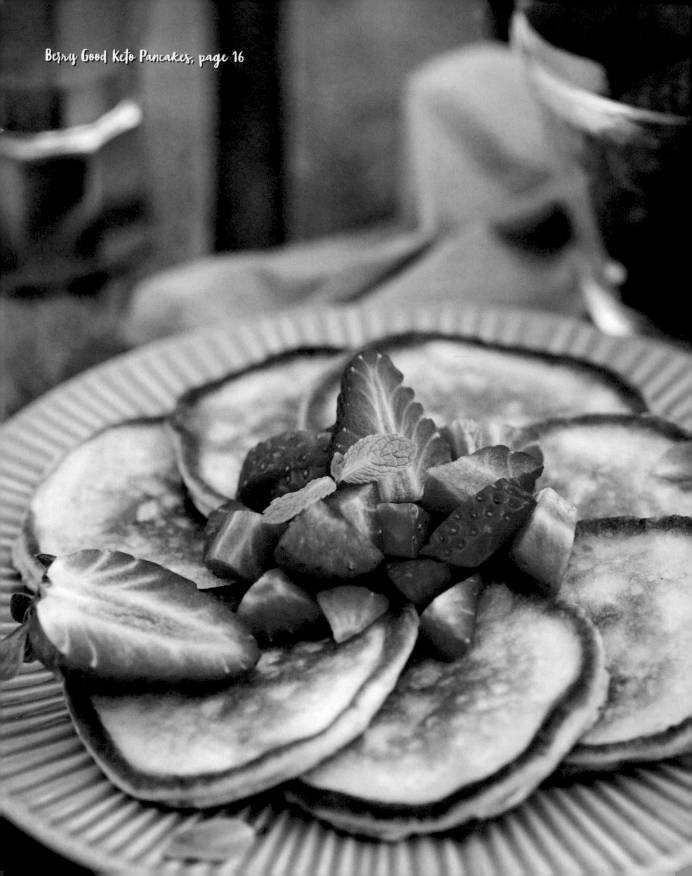

Berry Good Keto Pancakes, page 16

chapter 2
BREAKFASTS AND BRUNCHES

BERRY ALMOND FLAX SMOOTHIE

THIS SMOOTHIE IS A SNAP to put together for a quick and delicious on-the-go breakfast. Flaxseed oil, like fish oil, has long been studied for its heart-healthy benefits. Make sure to store it in the refrigerator, as this delicate oil can otherwise go bad quickly.

MAKES 2 SERVINGS

1 cup coconut milk

1 cup unsweetened almond milk

1 cup frozen berries

1 tablespoon flaxseed oil

2 teaspoons flaxseed

2 sprigs fresh mint

1 cup ice

Place the coconut milk, almond milk, berries, flaxseed oil, flaxseed, mint, and ice in a blender. Whirl the ingredients until smooth.

CALORIES 320 | PROTEIN 3 G (3%) | CARBS 14 G (15%) | FAT 33 G (82%) | SAT FAT 22 G FIBER 3 G

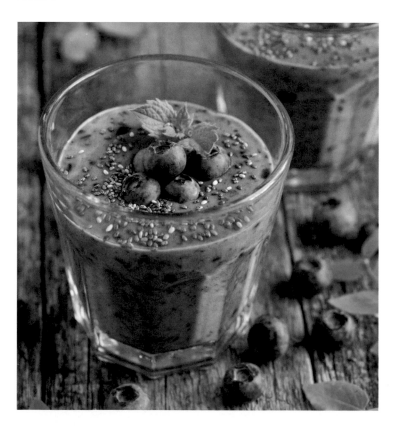

CHOCOLATE, PB, AND AVOCADO SMOOTHIE

THE MAGIC INGREDIENT in this smoothie mix: avocado. It's a simple (and creamy!) way to sneak a good amount of monounsaturated fats into your breakfast. These healthy fats are key nutrients in a ketogenic weight loss plan.

MAKES 2 SERVINGS

Place the chia seeds and ¼ cup water in a blender and let them sit for 10 minutes.

Add the coconut milk, avocado, peanut butter, cocoa powder, and ice. Whirl until the ingredients are smooth.

CALORIES 405 | PROTEIN 8 G (7%) | CARBS 15 G (14%) | FAT 38 G (79%) | SAT FAT 23.4 G
FIBER 8 G

1 tablespoon chia seeds

1 cup coconut milk

½ avocado, peeled

1 tablespoon smooth peanut butter

1 tablespoon cocoa powder

4 or 5 ice cubes

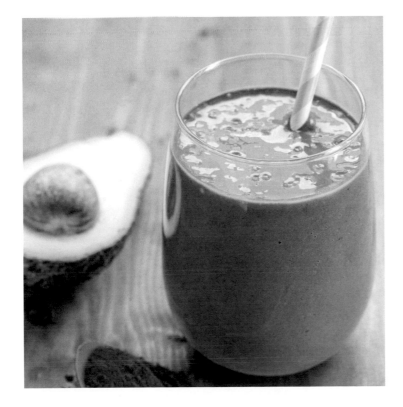

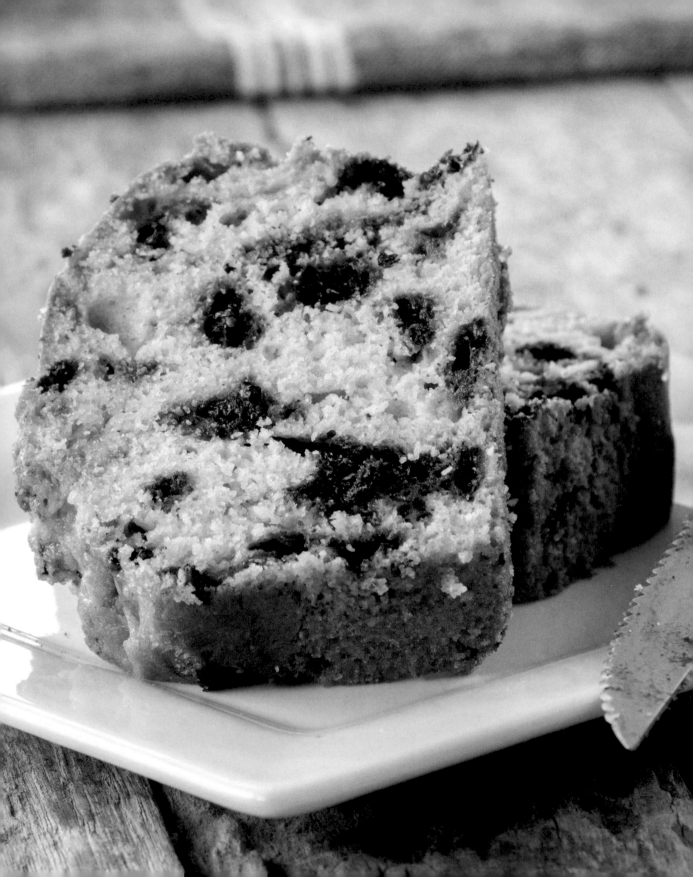

LEMON-BLUEBERRY BREAD

SWEET BLUEBERRIES AND TART LEMON zest are the perfect summertime pairing. But if fresh berries aren't available, frozen blueberries (or raspberries) make a very fine substitute. When lining the pan with parchment paper, let the paper hang slightly over the sides to form a "sling," which will make lifting the bread from the pan much easier.

MAKES 8 SERVINGS

Preheat the oven to 350°F. Brush a 9- x 5-inch baking pan with olive oil and line the bottom and long sides with a piece of parchment paper.

Combine the almond flour, baking soda, and salt in the work bowl of a food processor. Add the eggs, lemon juice, zest, vanilla extract, and stevia. Process until the ingredients are smooth. Stir in the blueberries and transfer the batter to the prepared pan.

Bake for 50 minutes or until a toothpick inserted into the center of the loaf comes out clean. Let the loaf cool to room temperature. Run a knife along the short ends of the pan and then hold the parchment to lift the bread out easily.

CALORIES 275 | PROTEIN 13 G (18%) | CARBS 11 G (15%) | FAT 21 G (67%)
SAT FAT 2.5 G | FIBER 5 G

3 cups almond flour

½ teaspoon baking soda

¼ teaspoon salt

6 large eggs + 1 egg white

2 teaspoons fresh lemon juice

Zest of 2 lemons

1 teaspoon vanilla extract

½ teaspoon liquid stevia

1 cup blueberries

BERRY GOOD KETO PANCAKES

FRESH STRAWBERRIES (or any substitute berries of your choice) take the place of syrup on these pancakes to lower the sugar and increase the fiber. There's no sacrifice in taste! Feeding a crowd? Simply double or triple the recipe.

MAKES 2 SERVINGS

3 tablespoons butter, divided

4 large eggs

4 ounces cream cheese

½ teaspoon vanilla extract

2 tablespoons vanilla whey protein powder

1 cup sliced strawberries

Place 2 tablespoons of the butter in a small microwavable bowl and microwave on HIGH for 30 seconds to melt. Combine the eggs, cream cheese, vanilla extract, protein powder, and melted butter in the work bowl of a food processor. Process the ingredients until smooth.

Heat the remaining tablespoon of butter in a large nonstick skillet over medium-high heat. When the skillet is hot, pour ¼ cup of the batter into the skillet. Repeat with the remaining batter. Cook the pancakes for 2 minutes until bubbles form and the pancakes begin to look dry on top. Flip them and cook for 1 minute longer. Serve them topped with sliced strawberries.

CALORIES 540 | PROTEIN 21 G (15%) | CARBS 10 G (7%) | FAT 47 G (78%)
SAT FAT 25 G | FIBER 2 G

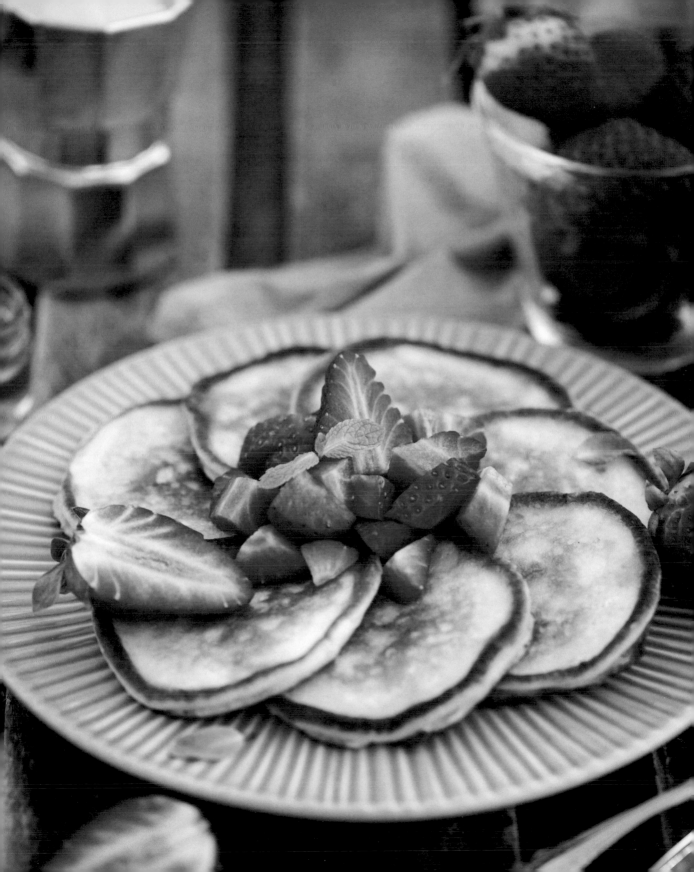

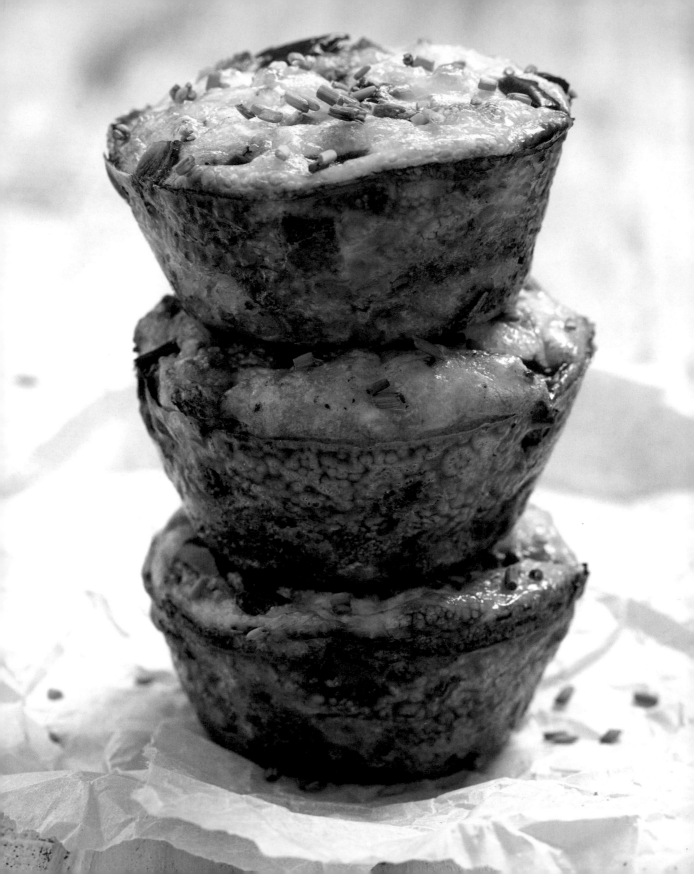

CHEESY HAM AND VEGGIE QUICHE CUPS

NOW YOU CAN TAKE QUICHE ON THE GO! These cups are perfect for a warm, cheesy egg breakfast even when you don't have time for a sit-down meal. Whip up a batch on a Sunday evening and you'll be set for days.

MAKES 6 SERVINGS

Preheat the oven to 350°F. Brush a 12-cup muffin tin with olive oil and set aside.

In a large bowl, whisk the eggs and season them with salt and pepper. Add the ham, onion, bell pepper, broccoli, and Cheddar. Stir the ingredients until thoroughly combined.

Distribute the mixture among the prepared muffin cups. Sprinkle the scallions on top. Bake for 20 minutes until the quiche cups are set and beginning to brown. Remove the tin from the oven and let the muffins cool for 10 minutes. Run a knife along the inside of each cup of the tin to loosen the muffins. If saving for later, let the muffins cool completely before refrigerating them.

CALORIES 295 | PROTEIN 23 G (32%) | CARBS 4 G (6%) | FAT 20 G (62%)
SAT FAT 9 G | FIBER 1 G

12 eggs

Salt and freshly ground black pepper

3 slices deli ham, sliced
(about ¾ cup)

¼ cup finely chopped onion

½ cup finely chopped bell pepper

1 cup finely chopped broccoli

1½ cups shredded Cheddar cheese

3 scallions, chopped

SAUSAGE AND ZUCCHINI FRITTATA

THIS SUPER-EASY FRITTATA is delicious for breakfast, brunch, any meal. Avoid using reduced-fat sausage. You'll notice this recipe doesn't call for extra oil, so the small amount of fat from the sausage is important for keeping this dish keto-friendly.

MAKES 4 SERVINGS

¼ pound bulk country breakfast sausage

2 cups sliced zucchini

Salt and freshly ground black pepper

6 scallions, thinly sliced

8 eggs, lightly beaten

1 cup shredded Provolone cheese

Preheat the oven to 425°F.

Cook the sausage in a large ovenproof skillet over medium-high heat for 5 to 6 minutes, breaking up the sausage with the side of a spoon as it cooks, until sausage is browned. Add the zucchini and cook another 5 minutes until it's softened. Season to taste with the salt and pepper. Stir in the scallions, and then pour the egg mixture on top. Cook another 2 to 3 minutes until the bottom begins to set.

Scatter the Provolone on top and bake for 7 to 9 minutes, until puffy and golden. Remove from the oven and let the frittata sit for a few minutes before serving.

CALORIES 300 | PROTEIN 23 G (31%) | CARBS 5 G (7%) | FAT 21 G (62%)
SAT FAT 9.2 G | FIBER 1 G

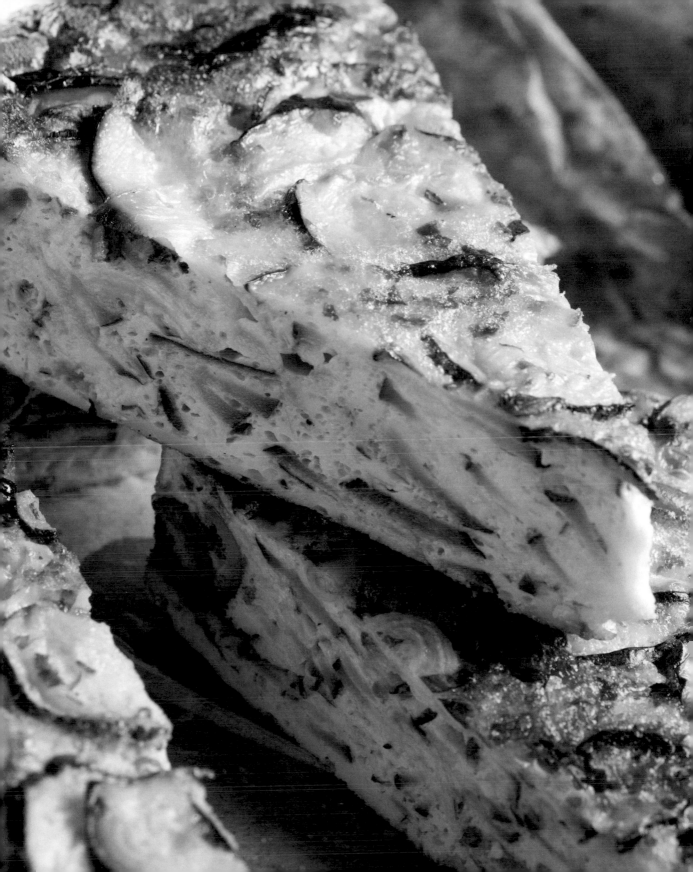

FRENCH OMELET *with Mushrooms*

MOST PEOPLE FIND THE RIND on a wheel of Brie, while still fresh, to be pleasant to eat. If it's not to your liking, simply cut it away and use the center portion of the cheese. Brie is amazingly rich and delicious in an omelet. Serve with fresh berries.

MAKES 1 SERVING

1 tablespoon butter

2 tablespoons finely chopped onion or shallot

½ cup sliced mushrooms

¼ teaspoon dried thyme

Salt and freshly ground black pepper

2 eggs, lightly beaten

1 ounce Brie cheese, sliced

Melt the butter in a 10-inch nonstick omelet pan over medium-high heat. Cook the onion or shallot for 1 to 2 minutes until it begins to soften. Add the mushrooms and thyme, and continue cooking for another 3 minutes until the mushrooms begin to look dry. Use a silicone spatula to distribute the mushrooms evenly across the pan. Season to taste with the salt and pepper.

Pour the eggs on top and immediately shake the pan until the egg mixture slips beneath the filling. Tilt the pan a few times so that the eggs extend slightly up the sides as they cook. When the omelet is set, arrange the Brie slices in the center. Use the spatula to gently fold the sides of the omelet over the Brie.

CALORIES 355 | PROTEIN 20 G (22%) | CARBS 4 G (5%) | FAT 29 G (73%)
SAT FAT 15.4 G | FIBER 1 G

CALIFORNIA EGGS BENEDICT

HOLLANDAISE SAUCE IS THE STAR of the show and extremely keto-friendly. Once you see how easy it is to make this sauce, you'll know it's not just for breakfast. Use it to top grilled asparagus or your favorite fish dish. If you miss the English muffin, the muffin recipe on page 24 makes a stellar replacement.

MAKES 2 SERVINGS

Fill a medium pot halfway with water and cook on high heat. When the water begins to simmer, reduce the heat to medium low and add 1 to 2 teaspoons of vinegar. Crack an egg into a small cup and gently slide it into the simmering water. Repeat with the remaining eggs. Poach the eggs for 2 minutes, then turn off the heat and let them cook another 10 minutes.

Meanwhile, melt the butter in a large skillet over medium-high heat. Add the spinach and cook it for 1 to 2 minutes until wilted. Season to taste with the salt and pepper. Arrange the tomato slices on the plates and then equal amounts of spinach. Use a slotted spoon to remove the poached eggs and place on the spinach. Spoon the hollandaise sauce on top and garnish with the parsley just before serving.

TO MAKE THE HOLLANDAISE SAUCE: Vigorously whisk the egg yolks and lemon juice in a double boiler over medium heat. Slowly stir in the butter, whisking until the sauce has doubled in volume. Season to taste with the cayenne and salt. Remove from the heat and cover to keep warm until ready to serve.

CALORIES 475 | PROTEIN 18 G (15%) | CARBS 6 G (5%) | FAT 43 G (80%)
SAT FAT 23 G | FIBER 2 G

1 to 2 teaspoons vinegar

4 eggs

1 tablespoon butter

4 cups spinach

Salt and freshly ground black pepper

4 large tomato slices (½-inch thick)

1 tablespoon fresh chopped parsley

Hollandaise Sauce

2 egg yolks

2 teaspoons fresh lemon juice

¼ cup butter, melted

Pinch of ground cayenne

¼ teaspoon salt

MUFFIN *in a Mug*

THESE VERSATILE, TASTY MUFFINS are super easy to make in small batches for those mornings when you crave a little bread with your breakfast. Another handy use: Toast them and use them as a base for the Eggs Benedict recipe you'll find on page 23.

MAKES 2 SERVINGS

3 tablespoons almond flour

1 tablespoon coconut flour

¼ teaspoon baking powder

Dash of salt

1 egg, lightly beaten

1 teaspoon olive oil

Brush the inside of a coffee mug with olive oil.

In a small bowl, combine the almond flour, coconut flour, baking powder, and salt. Add the egg and olive oil, and stir until the ingredients are thoroughly combined.

Transfer the batter to the mug, place in a microwave, and cook on HIGH for 1 minute. Slip a knife around the sides of the muffin so it slides out of the mug.

CALORIES 135 | PROTEIN 6 G (18%) | CARBS 3 G (9%) | FAT 11 G (73%)
SAT FAT 1.7 G | FIBER 2 G

HOMEMADE BREAKFAST SAUSAGE

MAKING UP A BATCH OF YOUR OWN breakfast sausage is a delicious and easy alternative to the store-bought stuff. Prepared breakfast sausage often comes loaded with additives and sodium that you're better off avoiding when you can. Double the recipe and freeze uncooked patties for up to three months. Skip the red pepper flakes if you don't enjoy spicy food.

MAKES 4 SERVINGS

In a large bowl, combine the pork, bacon fat, poultry seasoning, thyme, black pepper, and pepper flakes (if using). Mix the ingredients with clean hands until well combined. Form the mixture into 8 patties.

Meanwhile, warm a large nonstick skillet over medium-high heat. Fry the patties for 3 to 4 minutes per side until browned and the meat is cooked through.

CALORIES 285 | PROTEIN 23 G (30%) | CARBS 6 G (8%) | FAT 21 G (62%)
SAT FAT 7.5 G | FIBER 0 G

1 pound lean ground pork

1 tablespoon bacon fat

1 teaspoon poultry seasoning

½ teaspoon dried thyme

½ teaspoon freshly ground black pepper

½ teaspoon red pepper flakes (optional)

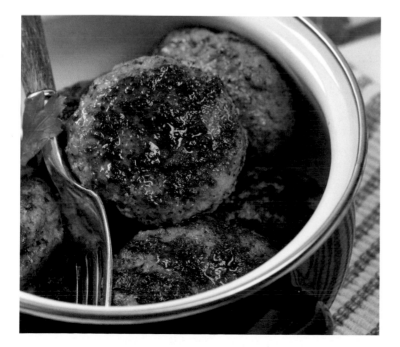

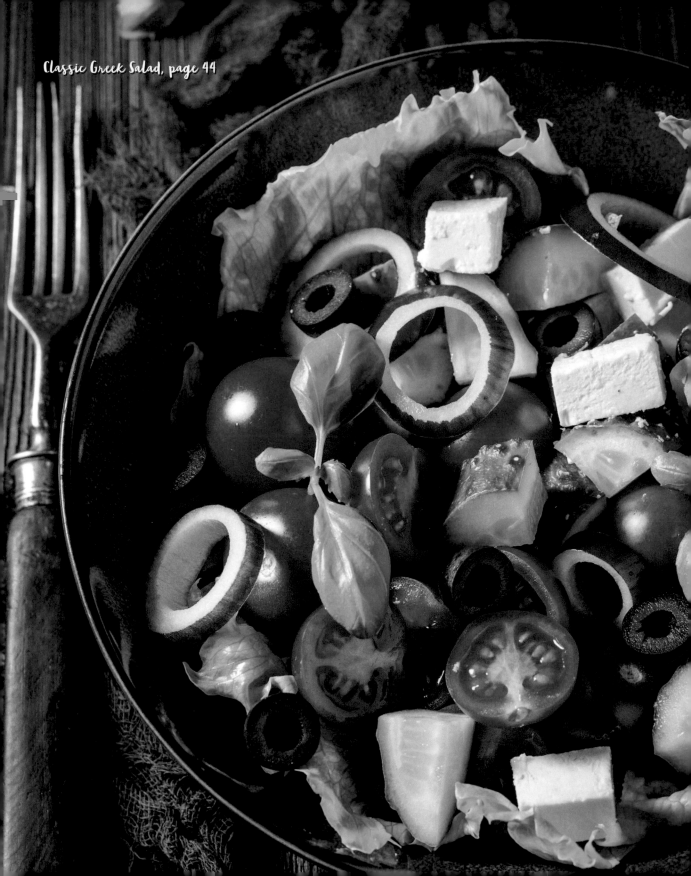

Classic Greek Salad, page 44

chapter 3
SANDWICHES, SOUPS, AND SALADS

EXTRA-CHEESY GRILLED CHEESE

THIS LUSCIOUS SANDWICH will take a big bite out of your carb allowance for the day, so plan accordingly. However, with 7 grams of fiber per serving, you're getting a healthy fiber boost, too.

1 head cauliflower florets, stems removed

1 large egg

½ cup shredded Parmesan cheese

1 teaspoon Italian herb seasoning

1 cup shredded Cheddar cheese

1 tomato, sliced

Preheat the oven to 450°F. Line a baking sheet with parchment paper.

Place the cauliflower into a food processor and pulse into fine crumbs about half the size of a grain of rice. Transfer the cauliflower into a large microwavable bowl, cover with a plate, and microwave on HIGH for 5 minutes, stopping to stir the cauliflower halfway through the cooking time so that it cooks evenly.

Allow the cauliflower to cool for a few minutes. Add the egg, Parmesan, and seasoning to the cauliflower and mix until thoroughly combined. Divide the mixture into 4 equal parts and transfer to the baking sheet. Shape the mixture into squares about ½-inch thick and bake for about 15 to 18 minutes or until golden brown. Remove from the oven and let them cool a few minutes.

Divide the Cheddar between 2 squares and top with the tomato slices. Using a good spatula, carefully slide the remaining squares off the parchment paper and place on top of the tomato slices. Bake the sandwiches for 5 to 10 minutes longer, until the cheese is completely melted.

CALORIES 455 | PROTEIN 30 G (25%) | CARBS 22 G (18%) | FAT 30 G (57%)
SAT FAT 16 G | FIBER 7 G

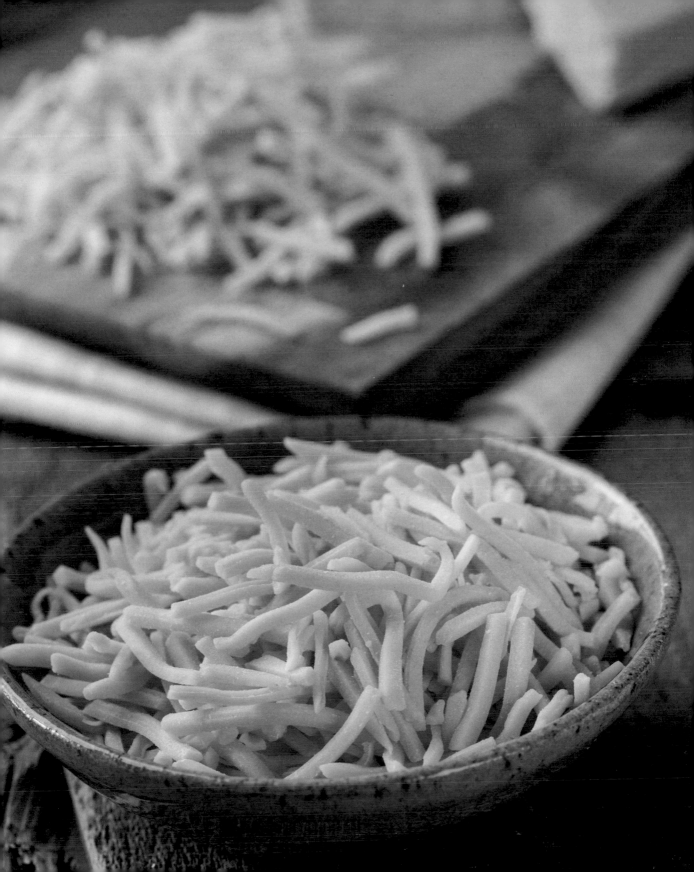

ITALIAN SUB LETTUCE ROLLUP

ENJOY ALL THE FLAVORS of your favorite sub-style sandwich wrapped up in a keto-friendly lettuce roll. You really will be hard-pressed to miss the bread. Make several to share and enjoy for a delicious picnic lunch.

MAKES 1 SERVING

1 large leaf lettuce

1 deli slice ham

1 slice Provolone cheese

3 deli slices hard salami

4 deli slices pepperoni

2 slices onion

5 or 6 slices pickled hot peppers

1 small Italian tomato, sliced

2 teaspoons olive oil

½ teaspoon balsamic vinegar

Dash of dried oregano

Trim the lettuce and lay it flat on a work surface. Layer the ham, Provolone, salami, and pepperoni slices on top. Add the onion, hot peppers, and tomato. Drizzle with olive oil and vinegar. Sprinkle with oregano. Roll up like a burrito to eat.

CALORIES 450 | PROTEIN 25 G (22%) | CARBS 7 G (6%) | FAT 36 G (72%)
SAT FAT 13.1 G | FIBER 1 G

KETO MONTE CRISTO SANDWICH

ULTRALOW-CARB PANCAKES take the place of the French toast traditionally featured in these sandwiches. If you don't have ricotta on hand, cottage cheese makes a great substitute.

MAKES 4 SERVINGS

Combine the eggs, ricotta, almond flour, salt, and baking soda in the work bowl of a blender. Whirl until the ingredients are smooth.

Heat the oil in a large nonstick skillet over medium-high heat. To make each pancake, ladle 2 tablespoons of batter at a time into the skillet. Tilt the skillet to spread the batter in a thin layer. Flip the pancake when it has stopped bubbling and begins to dry. Make a total of 8 pancakes.

To assemble the sandwiches, top one pancake with a few tablespoons of cheese, followed by a slice of ham and turkey and a few more tablespoons of cheese. Top with another pancake. Repeat with remaining ingredients until you have assembled 4 sandwiches.

Place the sandwiches back into the skillet over low heat. Cook for 2 to 3 minutes per side, until the cheese has melted. Drizzle with sugar-free syrup.

CALORIES 415 | PROTEIN 29 G (25%) | CARBS 24 G (20%) | FAT 29 G (55%)
SAT FAT 12.1 G | FIBER 3 G

3 eggs
½ cup ricotta cheese
½ cup almond flour
Pinch of salt
½ teaspoon baking soda
1 tablespoon coconut oil
4 slices deli ham
4 slices deli smoked turkey
1 cup shredded Swiss cheese
½ cup sugar-free syrup

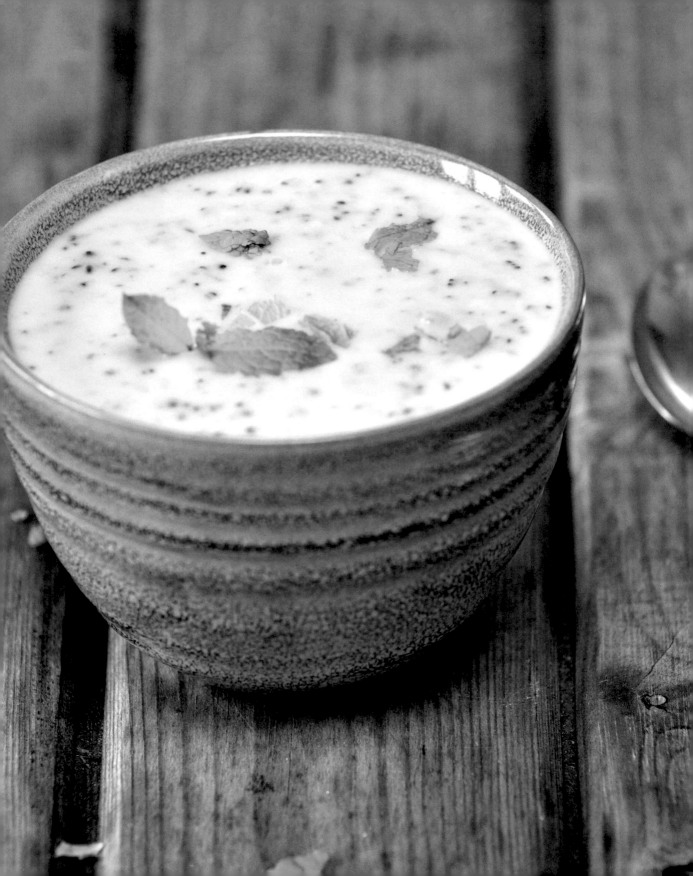

BROCCOLI-CHEDDAR SOUP

THINK OF THIS SOUP AS YOUR DAILY DOSE OF CREAMY, cheesy comfort food in a bowl. The broccoli adds a nice pop of color, as well as a bit of fiber.

MAKES 4 SERVINGS

In a large pot over medium heat, warm the oil and cook the garlic, stirring occasionally, for 1 to 2 minutes, until the garlic begins to brown. Add the florets, broth, and cream. Bring the soup to a boil and reduce the heat to low. Simmer for 10 minutes, until the broccoli is tender.

Using an immersion blender, puree the soup (alternately, use a food processor to process the soup in batches). Add the Cheddar, ½ cup at a time, and stir until melted. Season to taste with the salt and pepper.

CALORIES 425 | PROTEIN 21 G (20%) | CARBS 7 G (6%) | FAT 35 G (74%)
SAT FAT 18.7 G | FIBER 2 G

1 tablespoon olive oil

4 cloves garlic, chopped

½ pound broccoli crowns, chopped (about 6 cups)

4 cups reduced-sodium chicken broth

1 cup heavy cream

2 cups shredded Cheddar cheese

Salt and freshly ground black pepper

ITALIAN SAUSAGE AND KALE SOUP

THIS SOUP TRADITIONALLY INCLUDES WHITE BEANS, but in this keto-friendly version the addition of cauliflower florets makes a smart and tasty substitute.

MAKES 6 SERVINGS

1 pound sweet Italian sausage, casings removed

1 tablespoon butter

1 onion, chopped

2 cloves garlic, chopped

1 teaspoon dried oregano

½ teaspoon crushed red pepper flakes (optional)

4 cups reduced-sodium chicken broth

1 cup heavy whipping cream

2 cups chopped cauliflower florets

3 cups chopped kale

Salt and freshly ground black pepper

In a large pot over medium-high heat, cook the sausage for about 5 minutes until browned, using the side of a spoon to break up the meat as it cooks.

Transfer the sausage to a plate and discard the drippings, but do not wash the pot.

In the same pot, melt the butter over medium heat. Add the onion, garlic, oregano, and red pepper flakes (if using) and cook for 2 to 3 minutes, until the onions begin to soften. Add the broth and heavy cream. Scrape off any browned bits that have accumulated in the bottom of the pot. Increase the heat to medium high.

When the soup reaches a simmer, add the cauliflower, kale, and cooked sausage. Reduce the heat to medium low. Simmer for 10 minutes, until the cauliflower and kale are tender. Season to taste with the salt and pepper.

CALORIES 395 | PROTEIN 16 G (16%) | CARBS 6 G (6%) | FAT 34 G (78%)
SAT FAT 14.6 G | FIBER 2 G

SLOW-COOKER BUFFALO CHICKEN SOUP

HERE YOU'LL FIND ALL THE FLAVORS of your favorite sports bar snack food presented in a delicious bowl of soup. Plus, preparing a slow-cooker soup means it's easy to bring along to a potluck.

MAKES 4 SERVINGS

In a slow cooker, combine the onion and celery and place the chicken on top. Drizzle the ingredients with the butter and hot sauce. Add the broth. Cover and cook on HIGH for 3 hours or on LOW for 6 hours.

Move the chicken to a plate, shred it, and set it aside.

Add the cream and cream cheese and stir until the cheese is melted. Using an immersion blender, puree the soup until smooth. Season to taste with the salt and pepper. Add the chicken back into the soup. Top with scallions and additional hot sauce (if using) just before serving.

CALORIES 530 | PROTEIN 39 G (29%) | CARBS 5 G (4%) | FAT 40 G (67%)
SAT FAT 21.5 G | FIBER 1 G

½ onion, coarsely chopped

2 ribs celery, coarsely chopped

4 boneless, skinless chicken thighs (about 1½ pounds)

¼ cup butter, melted

¼ cup hot sauce, plus more for garnish

3 cups reduced-sodium chicken broth

1 cup heavy cream

4 ounces cream cheese, cut into 4 to 6 chunks

Salt and freshly ground black pepper

4 scallions, thinly sliced

SPICED PUMPKIN SOUP

SMART KETO CHOICES ARE ALL AROUND YOU. Make sure you use plain, unsweetened pumpkin for this recipe, not pumpkin pie filling, which is typically loaded with sugars you'll need to avoid. Don't worry: The natural flavors from the pumpkin, bacon, and spices will satisfy so much that you won't miss the added sugars!

MAKES 4 SERVINGS

4 slices center-cut bacon

2 tablespoons butter

½ onion, chopped

2 cloves garlic, minced

1½ teaspoons grated fresh ginger

¼ teaspoon ground cinnamon

¼ teaspoon ground nutmeg

1½ cups reduced-sodium chicken broth

1 cup pumpkin puree

½ cup heavy cream

Salt and freshly ground black pepper

In a large pot over medium-high heat, cook the bacon until crisp, about 5 minutes. Transfer the bacon to a plate lined with paper towels. When the bacon is cool, chop and set aside.

Add the butter, onion, and garlic to the pot and cook for 2 to 3 minutes until the onion is soft. Add the ginger, cinnamon, nutmeg, broth, and pumpkin. Stir the ingredients until thoroughly combined. Bring the soup to a boil and reduce the heat to low. Simmer for 20 minutes.

Using an immersion blender, puree the soup until smooth. Stir in the heavy cream and cook for 5 minutes longer to allow the flavors to combine. Season to taste with salt and pepper. Top with the reserved bacon just before serving.

CALORIES 265 | PROTEIN 7 G (10%) | CARBS 8 G (12%) | FAT 23 G (78%)
SAT FAT 11.1 G | FIBER 2 G

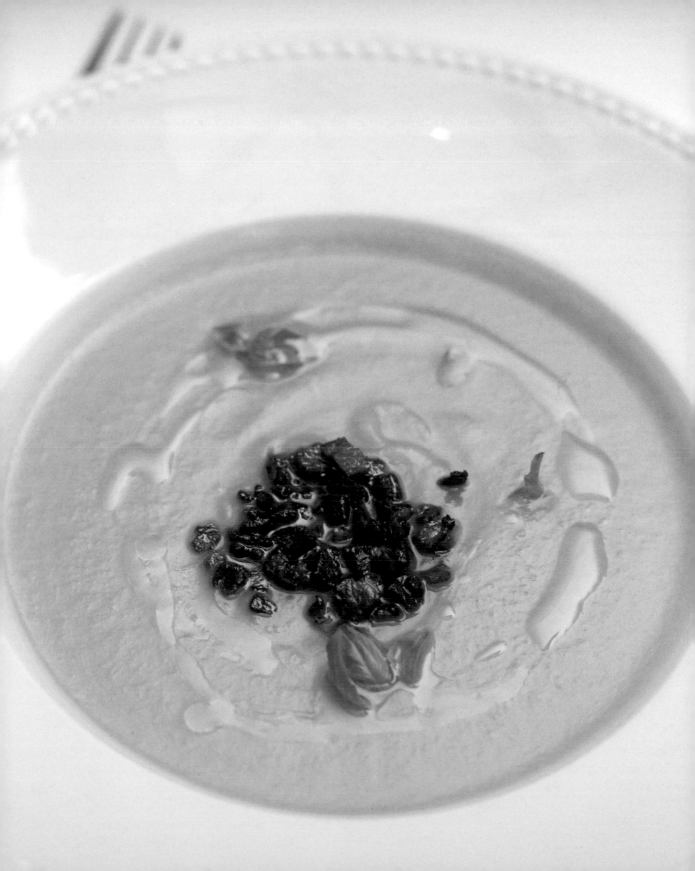

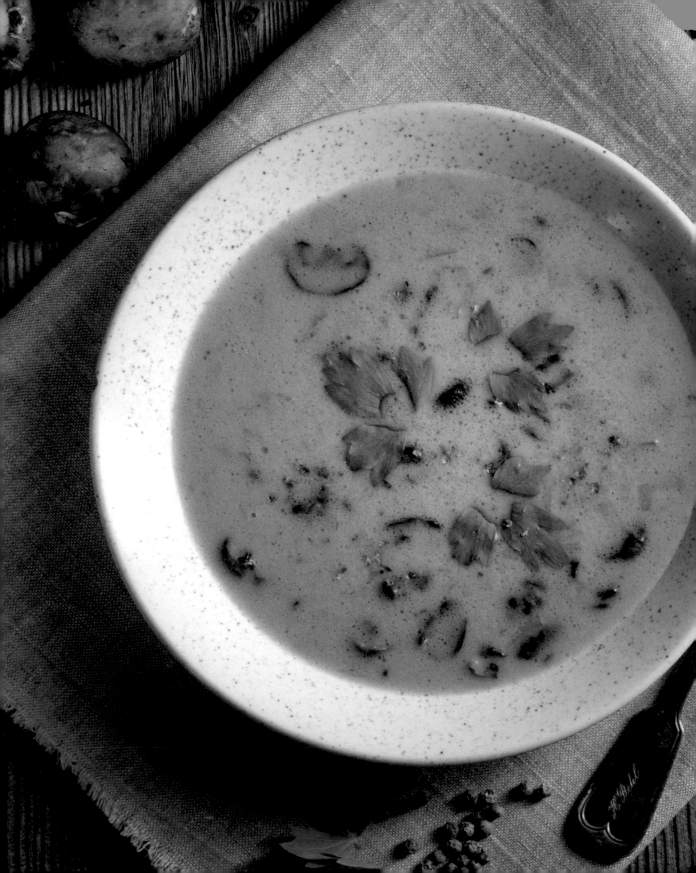

CREAMY MUSHROOM SOUP

SO MANY DELICIOUS KETO OPTIONS! For a vegetarian version of this soup, simply replace the chicken broth with vegetable stock. To save some prep time, buy presliced mushrooms if they're available. If you prefer a smooth consistency, use an immersion blender to puree the soup before adding the parsley.

MAKES 6 SERVINGS

In a large pot over medium-high heat, melt the butter. Add the mushrooms, onions, garlic, and thyme. Season to taste with the salt and pepper. Cook for 5 to 7 minutes, stirring occasionally, until the mushrooms are soft and the pot is beginning to look dry.

Add the chicken broth and scrape any brown bits that have accumulated on the bottom of the pot. Bring the soup to a boil and reduce the heat to low. Simmer for 20 minutes. Whisk in the cream cheese and heavy cream. Cook the soup 5 minutes longer until the cream cheese has melted and the soup is heated. Stir in the parsley just before serving.

CALORIES 300 | PROTEIN 8 G (10%) | CARBS 10 G (13%) | FAT 27 G (77%)
SAT FAT 16.1 G | FIBER 1 G

¼ cup butter

1½ pounds brown mushrooms, stemmed and sliced

1 onion, finely chopped

3 cloves garlic, minced

½ teaspoon dried thyme

Salt and freshly ground black pepper

4 cups reduced sodium chicken broth

2 ounces cream cheese

1 cup heavy cream

½ cup chopped fresh parsley

CREAMY CAULIFLOWER SOUP

CAULIFLOWER DOESN'T NEED TO BE BORING. Paired with celeriac, along with a hint of chives, this soup is brimming with flavor. If you prefer a smooth soup, simply puree the whole batch. To save a few minutes of prep time, feel free to use frozen cauliflower if you prefer.

MAKES 4 SERVINGS

¼ cup olive oil

4 cloves garlic, coarsely chopped

1 small head cauliflower florets, chopped

1 cup peeled and chopped celeriac

Salt and freshly ground black pepper

4 cups reduced-sodium chicken broth

1 cup heavy cream

1 tablespoon chopped chives

In a large pot, warm the oil over medium-high heat. Add the garlic and cook for 30 seconds or until fragrant. Add the cauliflower, celeriac, and broth. Bring to a boil and reduce the heat to low. Simmer for 30 minutes until the vegetables are soft. Using a slotted spoon, remove about 1 cup of the vegetables to a small bowl and set aside. Using an immersion blender, puree the soup. Stir in the heavy cream and let the soup simmer for another 5 minutes until heated. Stir in the chives and reserved vegetables just before serving.

CALORIES 410 | PROTEIN 8 G (8%) | CARBS 10 G (9%) | FAT 39 G (83%)
SAT FAT 16.4 G | FIBER 2 G

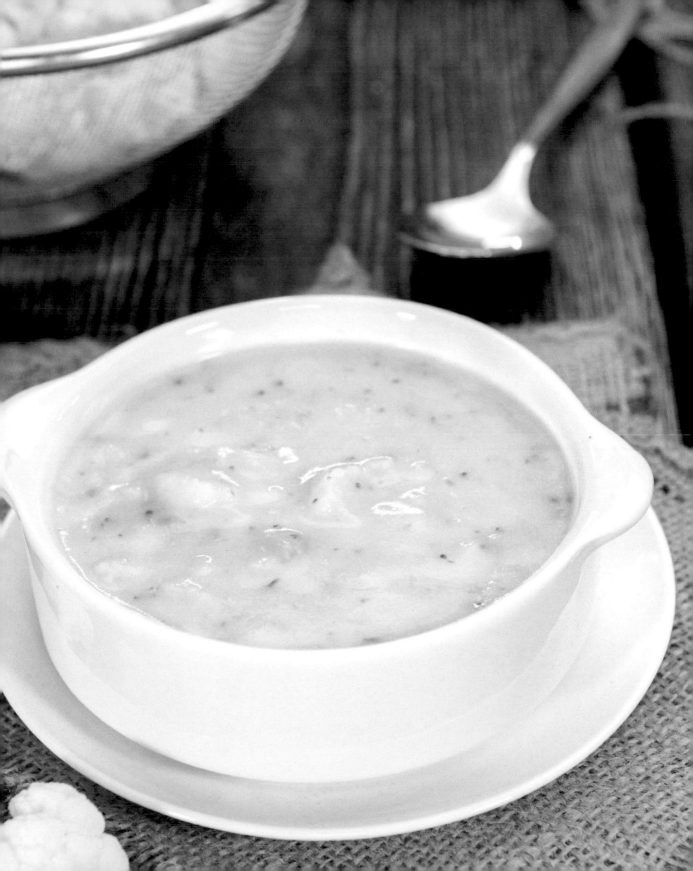

THAI SHRIMP SALAD

INSTEAD OF RELYING ON SUGAR (commonly found in many Thai dishes), this keto-friendly salad draws its natural sweetness from the onions, tomatoes, and bell pepper. Pre-cooked shrimp makes it so easy to put together.

MAKES 2 SERVINGS

¼ cup extra-virgin olive oil

2 tablespoons reduced-sodium soy sauce

1 teaspoon fish sauce

1 teaspoon chili garlic sauce

Juice of ½ lime

4 cups chopped romaine lettuce

½ pound cooked large shrimp, peeled

½ cup cherry tomatoes, halved

½ cup thinly sliced red bell pepper

¼ cup thinly sliced sweet onion

¼ cup chopped fresh cilantro

¼ cup finely chopped peanuts

2 tablespoons chopped fresh mint

In a large bowl, whisk together the olive oil, soy sauce, fish sauce, chili garlic sauce, and lime juice. Add the romaine, shrimp, tomatoes, bell pepper, and onion. Toss to coat. Top with the cilantro, peanuts, and fresh mint.

CALORIES 570 | PROTEIN 40 G (28%) | CARBS 17 G (12%) | FAT 39 G (60%)
SAT FAT 5.5 G | FIBER 6 G

SHRIMP AND AVOCADO SALAD

FRESH AND LIGHT YET SATISFYING, there are so many flavorful reasons to love this salad! To prepare an avocado easily, slice it in half, rolling it so that you cut around the stone. Twist the two halves to separate them and then use a spoon to remove the stone and scoop the flesh from the skin.

MAKES 2 SERVINGS

In a large bowl, whisk together the olive oil, lime juice, and cilantro. Season to taste with the salt and pepper. Add the spinach, romaine, shrimp, avocado, and onion. Toss gently to coat.

CALORIES 485 | PROTEIN 34 G (28%) | CARBS 14 G (11%) | FAT 34 G (61%)
SAT FAT 4.8 G | FIBER 7 G

2 tablespoons olive oil

Juice of ½ lime

½ cup chopped fresh cilantro

Salt and freshly ground black pepper

2 cups baby spinach

2 cups chopped romaine lettuce

½ pound cooked large shrimp, peeled

1 avocado, peeled and chopped

¼ cup thinly sliced sweet onion

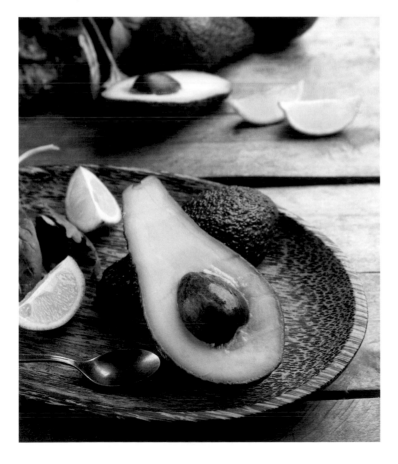

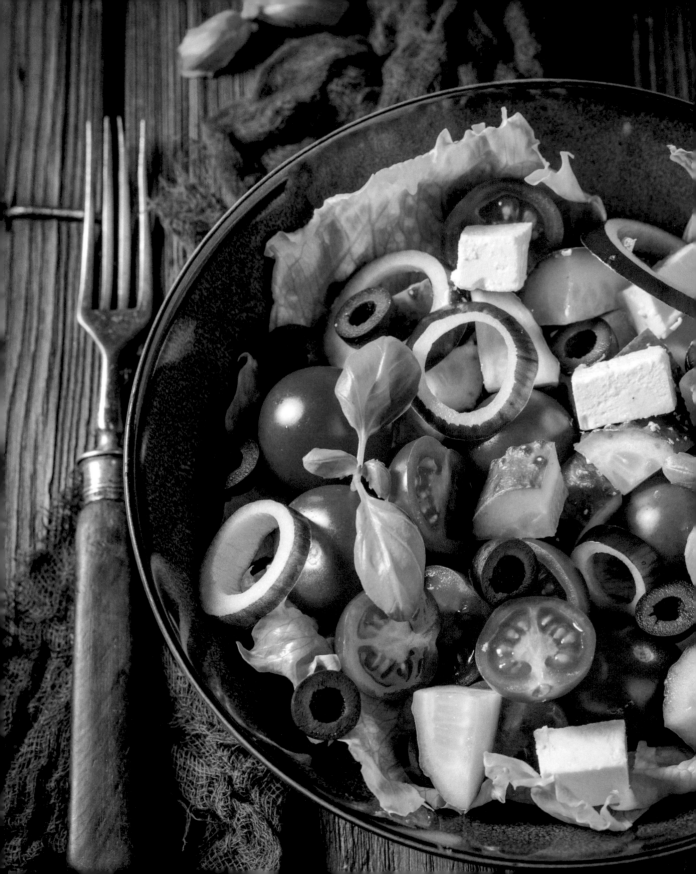

CLASSIC GREEK SALAD

WHEN MAKING GREEK SALAD, it's important to use a sturdy lettuce like romaine that will hold up to the strong flavors of the feta and olives. If you must find a replacement, avoid softer-leaved options like butter or Boston lettuce, which will become soggy rather quickly.

MAKES 2 SERVINGS

In a large bowl, whisk together the olive oil, vinegar, and oregano. Season to taste with the salt and pepper. Add the lettuce, tomato, cucumber, onion, feta, and olives. Toss to coat.

CALORIES 355 | PROTEIN 5 G (6%) | CARBS 11 G (12%) | FAT 33 G (82%)
SAT FAT 6.8 G | FIBER 4 G

¼ cup olive oil

2 tablespoons red wine vinegar

½ teaspoon dried oregano

Salt and freshly ground black pepper

3 cups chopped romaine lettuce

12 cherry tomatoes, halved

1 cup chopped cucumber

¼ cup thinly sliced red onion

¼ cup crumbled feta cheese

¼ cup black olives, chopped

KETO COBB SALAD

HAVE SOME LEFTOVER CHICKEN BREAST ON HAND? This colorful California salad is a cinch to put together. For a company-worthy arrangement, assemble the salad on a large platter and group the individual ingredients in rows or piles.

MAKES 4 SERVINGS

6 cups chopped romaine lettuce

2 cups chopped cooked skinless chicken breast

4 slices bacon, cooked and crumbled

4 hard-boiled eggs, sliced

1 large tomato, chopped

2 avocados, peeled and chopped

½ cup chopped Kalamata olives

¼ cup crumbled blue cheese

¼ cup olive oil

2 tablespoons red wine vinegar

2 tablespoons chopped fresh parsley

Salt and freshly ground black pepper

Place the romaine on a large platter (divide into 4 bowls if serving individually). Arrange the chicken, bacon, eggs, tomato, avocado, olives, and blue cheese on top. In a small bowl, whisk together the oil, vinegar, and parsley. Season to taste with the salt and pepper. Pour the dressing over the salad and serve.

CALORIES 535 | PROTEIN 35 G (26%) | CARBS 12 G (9%) | FAT 39 G (65%)
SAT FAT 8.5 G | FIBER 7 G

CRISPY TOFU AND BOK CHOY SALAD

WHEN YOU'RE CRAVING AN ALTERNATIVE to regular lettuce, turn to this hearty salad. It's super crunchy with a slightly bitter edge that nicely balances out all the other rich and spicy flavors.

MAKES 2 SERVINGS

Wrap the tofu in paper towels and put it on a baking sheet. Slide a plate under one side of the baking sheet so that it sits at an angle, and set a heavy skillet on top of the tofu. Allow it to drain for 30 minutes or up to an hour. Unwrap the tofu and cut it into 1-inch pieces.

Preheat the oven to 350°F. Line the baking sheet with parchment paper and place the tofu on the paper. Drizzle on 1 tablespoon of the soy sauce, the sesame oil, garlic, and vinegar. Toss gently to coat. Bake for 30 to 40 minutes, turning the pieces halfway through the cooking time, until the tofu is dry and beginning to form crisp edges.

In a large bowl, whisk together the remaining 2 tablespoons of the soy sauce, and the canola oil, chili garlic sauce, and peanut butter. Set it aside until you're ready to prepare the salad.

To assemble the salad, toss the bok choy and scallions with the dressing. Add the tofu and the lime juice. Toss again to coat. Sprinkle with the chia seeds just before serving.

CALORIES 490 | PROTEIN 27 G (20%) | CARBS 17 G (13%) | FAT 39 G (67%)
SAT FAT 4.2 G | FIBER 5 G

14 ounces extra-firm tofu

3 tablespoons reduced-sodium soy sauce, divided

1 tablespoon sesame oil

1 tablespoon minced garlic

1 tablespoon red wine vinegar

2 tablespoons canola oil

1 tablespoon chili garlic sauce

1 tablespoon smooth peanut butter

½ pound bok choy, chopped

2 scallions, chopped

Juice of ½ lime

1 tablespoon chia seeds

ITALIAN ARTICHOKE SALAD

WHILE YOU CAN BUY MARINATED ARTICHOKES, they are so much more flavorful if you prepare and marinate them yourself. Tossed with olives, peppers, and fresh mozzarella cheese, serve this salad at room temperature on a bed of crunchy romaine. You will enjoy all your favorite Italian flavors with a generous amount of fiber.

MAKES 2 SERVINGS

1 tablespoon fresh lemon juice

1 teaspoon salt

6 baby artichokes

¼ cup olive oil

1 tablespoon capers, drained

¼ cup chopped Kalamata olives

¼ cup jarred cherry peppers, halved

2 teaspoons balsamic vinegar

2 cloves garlic, minced

½ teaspoon dried oregano

3 cups chopped romaine lettuce

2 ounces fresh mozzarella cheese, chopped

Fill a pot with about 6 cups of water. Add the lemon juice and salt.

Trim the tough outer leaves from the artichokes and cut them in half lengthwise. Spoon out the hairy center, leaving as much of the smooth white heart as possible. Trim the stems to about 1 inch, and cut off any stringy outer parts. Place the artichokes in the pot of water as soon as they are trimmed. Bring the water to a boil and reduce the heat. Simmer for 20 to 30 minutes, until the artichokes are fork tender.

In a large bowl, whisk together the olive oil, capers, olives, peppers, vinegar, garlic, and oregano. Drain the artichokes and add them to the dressing while they are still warm. Toss gently to coat. Let the artichokes sit for at least 10 minutes to cool and allow flavors to combine. Toss with the romaine and fresh mozzarella before serving.

CALORIES 425 | PROTEIN 11 G (10%) | CARBS 19 G (17%) | FAT 36 G (73%)
SAT FAT 7.6 G | FIBER 10 G

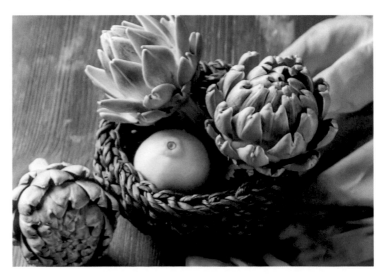

BLACKENED CHICKEN AND AVOCADO SALAD

USE A CAST-IRON SKILLET, if you have one, to cook the chicken. Alternately, if you prefer to grill the chicken, just make sure to add 4 tablespoons of oil to your dressing instead of dividing it. Those monounsaturated fats keep this salad keto-friendly.

MAKES 4 SERVINGS

In a small bowl, combine the paprika, garlic powder, chili powder, and cumin in a small bowl. Sprinkle the mixture over the chicken and rub to coat. Season to taste with the salt and pepper.

In a large, heavy skillet, warm 1 tablespoon of the oil over medium-high heat. Cook the chicken for 8 minutes per side, until the temperature in the center registers 165°F. Transfer the chicken to a plate and let it cool for 10 minutes before chopping.

In a large bowl, whisk together the remaining 3 tablespoons of oil and the lemon juice. Add the romaine, avocado, tomato, cucumber, onion, and chopped chicken. Toss to coat.

CALORIES 400 | PROTEIN 28 G (28%) | CARBS 12 G (12%) | FAT 27 G (60%)
SAT FAT 4 G | FIBER 7 G

½ teaspoon paprika

½ teaspoon garlic powder

½ teaspoon chili powder

½ teaspoon ground cumin

1 pound boneless, skinless chicken breasts

Salt and freshly ground black pepper

4 tablespoons olive oil, divided

Juice of ½ lemon

4 cups chopped romaine lettuce

2 avocados, peeled and chopped

1 large tomato, chopped

1 cup chopped cucumber

½ cup thinly sliced red onion

CURRIED CHICKEN SALAD

YOU CAN CERTAINLY USE POACHED CHICKEN BREASTS in this recipe if you prefer, but here you'll find roasting instructions; in general roasting intensifies flavor, which works well in a spicy curry dish. For a more colorful presentation, top with cherry tomato halves or chopped cucumber.

MAKES 4 SERVINGS

2 large bone-in chicken breast halves, about 1½ pounds

2 teaspoons olive oil

Salt and freshly ground black pepper

½ cup chopped celery

½ cup mayonnaise

1 teaspoons curry powder

Juice of ½ lemon

2 scallions, thinly sliced

4 cups chopped romaine lettuce

½ cup chopped cashews

½ cup cherry tomato halves (optional)

½ cup chopped cucumber (optional)

Preheat the oven to 350°F.

Place the chicken breasts on a baking sheet, rub the skin with olive oil, and sprinkle it generously with salt and pepper. Roast the chicken for 35 to 40 minutes, until the internal temperature reaches 165°F. Transfer the chicken to a plate and let it cool. Remove the meat from the bones, discard the skin, and chop the chicken into large bite-size pieces.

In a large bowl, combine the chicken, celery, mayonnaise, curry powder, lemon juice, and scallions. Mix gently until thoroughly combined. Season to taste with the salt and pepper. Serve on a bed of romaine topped with the cashews. Garnish with the cherry tomatoes or cucumbers (if using).

CALORIES 411 | PROTEIN 19 G (18%) | CARBS 10 G (9%) | FAT 34 G (73%)
SAT FAT 5.7 G | FIBER 2 G

FENNEL-WALNUT CHICKEN SALAD

POACHED CHICKEN BREASTS ARE EASY to make and result in exceptionally tender, moist meat, a perfect complement in this light, crunchy salad. Freeze the leftover broth in 1-cup containers; toss into a quick soup for another super-fast weeknight meal.

MAKES 4 SERVINGS

Place the chicken in a pot just large enough to hold the chicken breast halves and cover them with 1 inch of water. Add the bay leaf and a generous amount of salt and pepper. Bring to a simmer over medium-high heat just to the point when bubbles start forming around the edge of the pot. Reduce heat to medium low, letting the bubbles continue at a slow, steady rate. Cook the chicken, occasionally skimming foam from the water surface, for 15 to 18 minutes, until the internal temperature reaches 165°F. Discard the bay leaf.

Transfer the chicken to a heatproof bowl and let the chicken breasts cool. Reserve the resulting broth and refrigerate it until ready for use, up to 3 days. Remove the meat from the bones and cut it into bite-size pieces.

In a large bowl, combine the chicken, fennel, celery, walnuts, mayonnaise, walnut oil, lemon juice, and fennel fronds. Mix gently until thoroughly combined. Season to taste with the salt and pepper. Serve on a bed of arugula.

CALORIES 525 | PROTEIN 41 G (31%) | CARBS 5 G (4%) | FAT 38 G (65%)
SAT FAT 5.4 G | FIBER 2 G

2 large bone-in, skinless chicken breast halves, about 1½ pounds

1 bay leaf

Salt and freshly ground black pepper

1 cup fresh fennel, coarsely chopped

½ cup chopped celery

¼ cup toasted walnuts, chopped

½ cup mayonnaise

2 tablespoons walnut oil

Juice of ½ lemon

2 tablespoons chopped fennel fronds

4 cups baby arugula

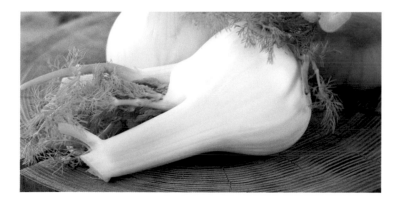

SPINACH, BLUE CHEESE, AND BACON SALAD

TOASTED NUTS MAKE A STATEMENT in a salad. To prepare them on the stovetop, simply cook the nuts in a dry skillet over medium-high heat for about 5 minutes, until fragrant. In the last minute or two, keep the nuts moving in the skillet. They can easily go from deliciously toasted to burnt in a matter of seconds.

MAKES 2 SERVINGS

3 tablespoons olive oil

1 tablespoon balsamic vinegar

Salt and freshly ground black pepper

4 cups baby spinach

½ cup thinly sliced red onion

¼ cup crumbled blue cheese

¼ cup chopped pecans, toasted

4 slices cooked bacon, chopped

In a large bowl, whisk together the olive oil and vinegar. Season to taste with the salt and pepper. Add the spinach, onion, blue cheese, pecans, and bacon. Toss to coat.

CALORIES 450 | PROTEIN 13 G (15%) | CARBS 9 G (10%) | FAT 30 G (75%)
SAT FAT 9 G | FIBER 3 G

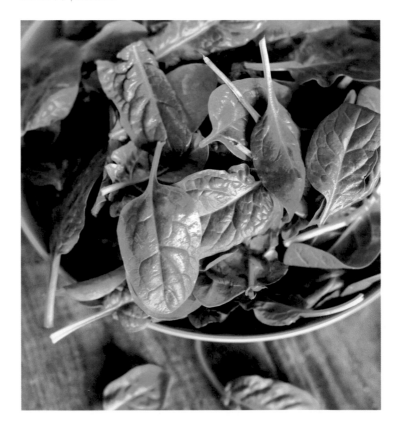

BEEF FAJITA SALAD

DON'T LET THE NUMBER OF INGREDIENTS dissuade you. This tender beef salad is made in your slow cooker, so you don't heat up your kitchen. It's a perfect fix-it-and-forget-it solution should you crave a hearty salad on a hot summer day!

MAKES 6 SERVINGS

Warm 1 tablespoon of oil in a large skillet over medium-high heat. Season the beef with salt and pepper. Cook, in batches if necessary, for 10 minutes until browned. Transfer the beef to a slow cooker. Add the diced tomatoes (with juice), onion, celery, bay leaf, chili powder, cumin, and garlic powder. Stir until thoroughly combined. Cover and cook on HIGH for 6 hours until the beef is fork tender. Transfer the beef to a plate and let the beef cool to room temperature before assembling the salad.

In a large bowl, whisk together the remaining ⅓ cup olive oil, lime juice, and cilantro. Season to taste with the salt and pepper. Add the cabbage, Cheddar, avocado, cherry tomatoes, bell pepper, and onion. Toss to coat. Top with the beef and 1 tablespoon of sour cream per serving.

CALORIES 515 | PROTEIN 41 G (31%) | CARBS 14 G (11%) | FAT 34 G (58%)
SAT FAT 10 G | FIBER 6 G

1 tablespoon + ⅓ cup olive oil, divided

2 pounds beef chuck, trimmed and cut into 1-inch pieces

Salt and freshly ground black pepper

1 can (14.5-ounce) diced tomatoes

1 onion, coarsely chopped

2 ribs celery, coarsely chopped

1 bay leaf

1 tablespoon chili powder

1 teaspoon ground cumin

1 teaspoon garlic powder

Juice of ½ lime

½ cup chopped fresh cilantro

6 cups shredded cabbage

1 cup shredded Cheddar cheese

1 avocado, peeled and chopped

1 cup cherry tomato halves

½ yellow bell pepper, sliced

½ sweet onion, sliced

6 tablespoons sour cream

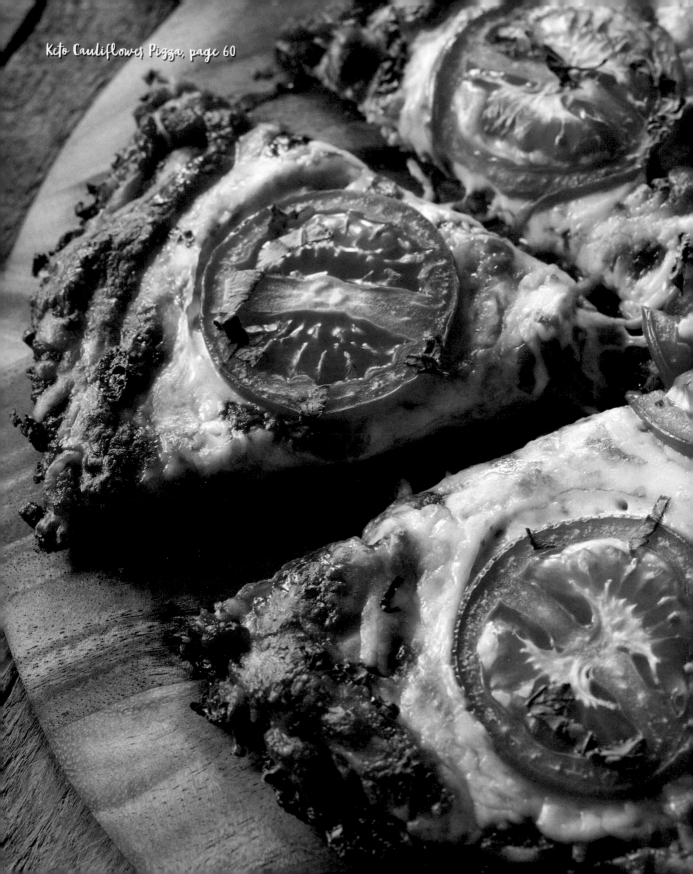
Keto Cauliflower Pizza, page 60

chapter 4

MAIN DISHES

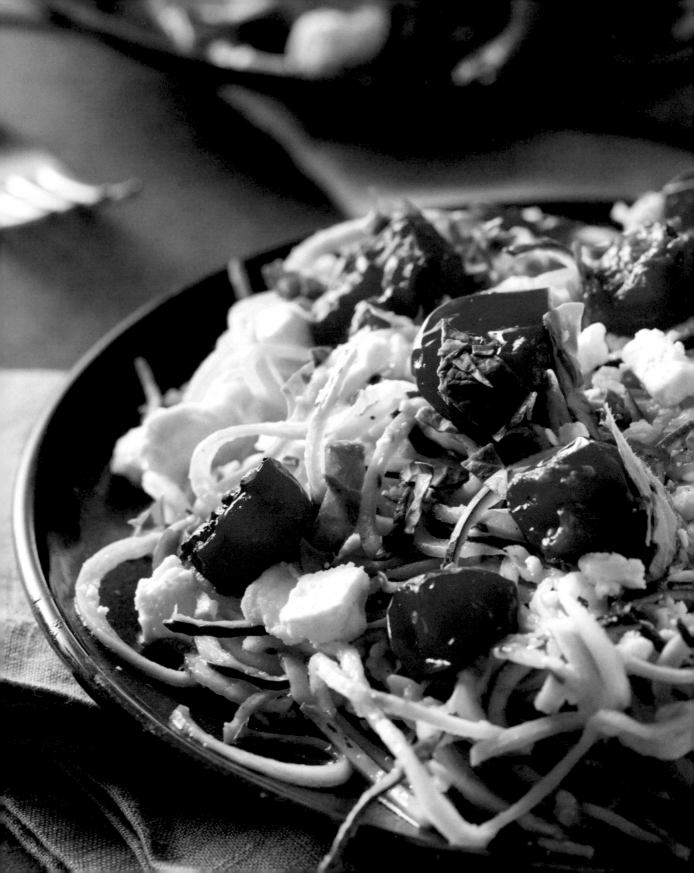

VERY VEGGIE PASTA "NOODLES"

YOU CAN TRANSFORM MANY DIFFERENT VEGETABLES INTO DELICIOUS, low-carb noodles in seconds with a spiralizer tool. For best results, look for vegetables that are at least 2 inches in diameter and relatively straight, though you can, of course, trim as necessary to get the ideal shape.

MAKES 2 SERVINGS

In a large skillet, warm the oil over medium-high heat. Add the garlic and cook for 30 seconds until fragrant.

Add the tomatoes. Cook for 3 to 5 minutes, stirring often, until the tomatoes soften and begin to release their juices. Season to taste with the salt and pepper.

Add the zucchini and squash noodles. Cover and cook for 2 to 3 minutes until the noodles are tender.

Add the lemon juice, feta, and basil. Toss to coat.

CALORIES 215 | PROTEIN 7 G (12%) | CARBS 12 G (21%) | FAT 17 G (67%)
SAT FAT 5.7 G | FIBER 3 G

3 tablespoons olive oil

3 cloves garlic, minced

1 pint cherry or grape tomatoes, halved

Salt and freshly ground black pepper

1 large zucchini, trimmed and spiralized into thick noodles

1 large yellow squash, trimmed and spiralized into thick noodles

Juice of ½ lemon

4 ounces feta cheese, crumbled (about 1 cup)

¼ cup chopped fresh basil

SPAGHETTI SQUASH
with Walnut Pesto

THINK OF SPAGHETTI SQUASH AS MOTHER NATURE'S PASTA. It separates easily into strands and holds the delicious walnut pesto just as nicely as regular spaghetti—but without all the extra carbs.

MAKES 8 SERVINGS

1 medium spaghetti squash, halved and seeded

3 tablespoons olive oil, divided

Salt and freshly ground black pepper

1 red bell pepper, finely chopped

1 onion, finely diced

1 cup prepared basil pesto

1 cup toasted walnuts

Shredded Parmesan cheese (optional)

Preheat the oven to 400°F. Line a baking sheet with parchment paper. Brush it with olive oil.

Use a fork to poke the skin of the spaghetti squash, and rub both sides with 1 tablespoon oil. Season to taste with salt and pepper.

Arrange the squash halves, cut-side down on the baking sheet, and bake for 40 to 45 minutes or until the squash is tender. Flip the halves so they're cut-side up and let them sit until they are cool enough to handle. Use a fork to shred the squash by drawing across the flesh to separate it into strands. Transfer the squash to a large bowl. Set aside.

In a large skillet, heat the remaining 2 tablespoons of oil over medium-high heat. Cook the bell pepper and onion until lightly golden, about 5 to 7 minutes. Add the reserved spaghetti squash and pesto to the skillet and cook, stirring occasionally, for 1 to 2 minutes longer until the squash is heated through. Adjust the seasonings and top with the walnuts and Parmesan (if using).

CALORIES 350 | PROTEIN 6 G (7%) | CARBS 13 G (14%) | FAT 32 G (79%)
SAT FAT 4.7 G | FIBER 4 G

SCALLION PANCAKES
with Spicy Mushrooms

THESE PANCAKES ARE THICK, so they don't fold like scallion pancakes you'd find in a dim sum shop. However, they're light and very filling. And with 4 grams of fiber per serving, they are well worth the slightly higher carb values.

MAKES 4 SERVINGS

TO MAKE THE MUSHROOMS: In a large skillet, heat the sesame oil over high heat. Add the mushrooms, ginger, soy sauce, and chili garlic sauce (if using). Cook, stirring occasionally, until the mushrooms are browned and the skillet begins to dry, about 5 minutes. Remove the skillet from the heat. Taste and adjust the seasonings. Set aside.

TO MAKE THE PANCAKES: Finely chop the cauliflower florets in a food processor. Transfer the cauliflower to a large microwavable bowl and cover with a plate. Microwave on HIGH for about 3 minutes. Let the cauliflower stand for another 3 minutes.

Finely chop the scallions and onion in the food processor. Add the onion mix to the cauliflower and stir to combine. Stir in the eggs and salt until the mixture is thoroughly combined.

In an omelet pan, working in batches, heat 1 tablespoon of the coconut oil over medium-high heat. Pour ¼ of the cauliflower mixture into the pan and use a spatula to spread it evenly. Cook it for 3 minutes until the bottom is set. Slide the pancake onto a plate. Cover with another plate and flip it. Slide the pancake, now cooked-side up, back into the pan and continue cooking another 3 minutes until browned on both sides and cooked through. Transfer the pancake to a plate and repeat with the remaining ingredients. Top the pancakes with the mushrooms.

CALORIES 310 | PROTEIN 19 G (23%) | CARBS 17 G (20%) | FAT 21 G (57%)
SAT FAT 9.7 G | FIBER 4 G

Mushrooms

1 tablespoon toasted sesame oil

1 pound mushrooms, preferably brown or shitake, stemmed and sliced

1 tablespoon grated fresh ginger

1 tablespoon reduced-sodium soy sauce

1½ teaspoons chili garlic sauce (optional)

Pancakes

1 head cauliflower florets

12 scallions

¼ cup chopped onion

8 eggs, lightly beaten

½ teaspoon salt

2 tablespoons coconut oil

KETO CAULIFLOWER PIZZA

HERE'S AN INTERESTING TAKE on an American classic. Loaded with Italian flavors, this pizza crust is held together with eggs and cheese, so it's gluten-free *and* keto-friendly.

MAKES 4 SERVINGS

1 head cauliflower florets

2 cups shredded mozzarella cheese, divided

¼ cup + 2 tablespoons grated Parmesan cheese, divided

1 large egg

½ teaspoon salt

1½ teaspoons garlic powder

1½ teaspoons dried oregano

½ cup no-sugar-added marinara sauce

2 Roma tomatoes, thinly sliced

1 tablespoon olive oil

Preheat the oven to 425°F. Line a baking sheet with parchment paper. Brush it with olive oil.

Finely chop the cauliflower florets in a food processor. Transfer the cauliflower to a large microwavable bowl and cover with a plate. Microwave on HIGH for about 3 minutes. Place the cauliflower on a clean towel, draw up the sides, and squeeze tightly over a sink to remove the excess moisture. Return the cauliflower to the bowl and add 1 cup of mozzarella, ¼ cup of the Parmesan, the egg, salt, garlic powder, and oregano. Stir until thoroughly combined.

Transfer the mixture to the baking sheet and pat gently into a thin, flat disc about 13 inches in diameter to form the pizza crust. Use a paper towel to blot any moisture on top of the crust. Bake for 15 minutes until it begins to brown. Let cool for 5 minutes, and blot any more moisture that has accumulated on top. Place a second sheet of parchment paper over the crust, and holding the edges of both sheets together, carefully lift the crust off the baking sheet, flip it, and place it back on the baking sheet. The new sheet of parchment paper is now on the bottom. Remove the top piece of paper and bake the crust for another 5 to 10 minutes until the top begins to brown.

Remove the crust from the oven. Spread the tomato sauce on top, followed by the remaining cup of mozzarella and the tomato slices. Bake for 5 to 10 minutes longer, until the cheese is melted and beginning to brown. Remove the pizza from the oven and let it sit for 10 minutes before cutting into slices. Sprinkle the remaining 2 tablespoons of Parmesan on top and drizzle on the olive oil before serving.

CALORIES 310 | PROTEIN 22 G (28%) | CARBS 15 G (19%) | FAT 19 G (54%)
SAT FAT 9.6 G | FIBER 4 G

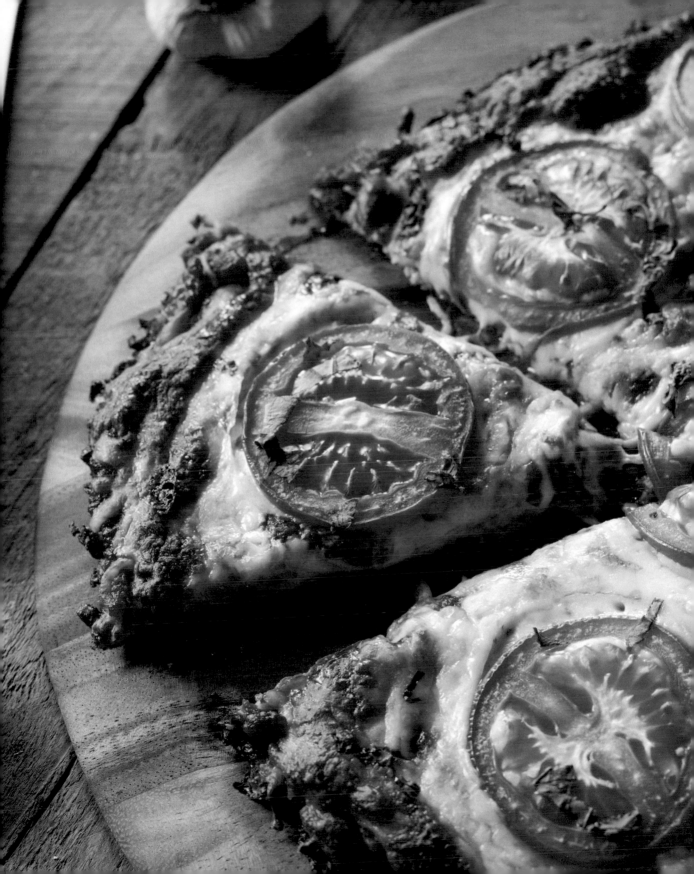

STUFFED PORTABELLA PIZZA

HERE'S ANOTHER LOWER-CARB PIZZA option that's super satisfying. If you're not a basil pesto fan, try sun-dried tomato pesto instead. The fat content of the pesto is key to keeping this dish keto-friendly. To save prep time, stock on up roasted peppers from your grocery's olive bar, or look for them in jars in the Italian section of your market.

MAKES 4 SERVINGS

4 large portabella mushrooms

2 tablespoons olive oil

Salt and freshly ground black pepper

½ cup prepared pesto

6 ounces fresh mozzarella cheese, chopped

½ cup roasted bell pepper strips

Preheat the broiler. Line a broiling pan with aluminum foil.

Remove the mushroom stems and use the side of a spoon to carefully scrape the gills from the underside of the mushrooms. Drizzle on the oil, rubbing the mushrooms to ensure they're evenly coated. Season to taste with the salt and pepper.

Arrange them smooth-side up on a broiling pan and broil for 4 to 5 minutes until the edges begin to brown. Flip the mushrooms and broil 3 to 4 minutes longer.

Remove the mushrooms from the broiler, spread the pesto evenly on each (about 2 tablespoons per mushroom), and top with equal amounts of mozzarella and pepper strips. Broil for 2 to 3 minutes longer, until cheese is melted and beginning to bubble.

CALORIES 355 | PROTEIN 16 G (18%) | CARBS 7 G (7%) | FAT 30 G (75%)
SAT FAT 9 G | FIBER 2 G

BAKED MANICOTTI CREPES

THESE TENDER CREPES are so easy to make. Filled with creamy ricotta and topped with tomato sauce, they make a very satisfying alternative to lasagna. If fresh basil isn't easily available, use spinach and add ½ teaspoon of dried basil to the cheese mixture.

MAKES 4 SERVINGS

Preheat the oven to 375°F. Brush an 8- x 8-inch baking dish with olive oil.

In the work bowl of a blender, whirl 4 eggs, the cream, garlic powder, and ½ teaspoon of salt until the ingredients are smooth. In a 10-inch skillet, melt about 1 teaspoon of butter over medium-high heat. Working in batches, pour about 2 tablespoons of the egg mixture into the skillet and tilt it so that batter evenly coats the bottom. Cook until the top is set. Transfer it to a plate and repeat with the remaining ingredients (you should have 8 crepes).

In a bowl, mix the ricotta, basil, the remaining egg, and ½ teaspoon of salt. Stir until thoroughly combined.

Pour about ¼ cup of the marinara into the bottom of the baking dish. Take a crepe, spread 2 tablespoons of the ricotta mixture in the center, and roll it up, placing it seam-side down in the baking dish. Repeat with the other crepes. Pour the remaining ¼ cup of marinara over the crepes and top with the mozzarella. Bake for 15 minutes until heated through.

CALORIES 415 | PROTEIN 23 G (22%) | CARBS 10 G (10%) | FAT 32 G (68%)
SAT FAT 17.7 G | FIBER 1 G

5 eggs, divided

¼ cup heavy cream

½ teaspoon garlic powder

1 teaspoon salt, divided

3 tablespoons butter

1 cup ricotta cheese

½ cup chopped fresh basil

½ cup no-sugar-added marinara sauce

1 cup shredded mozzarella cheese

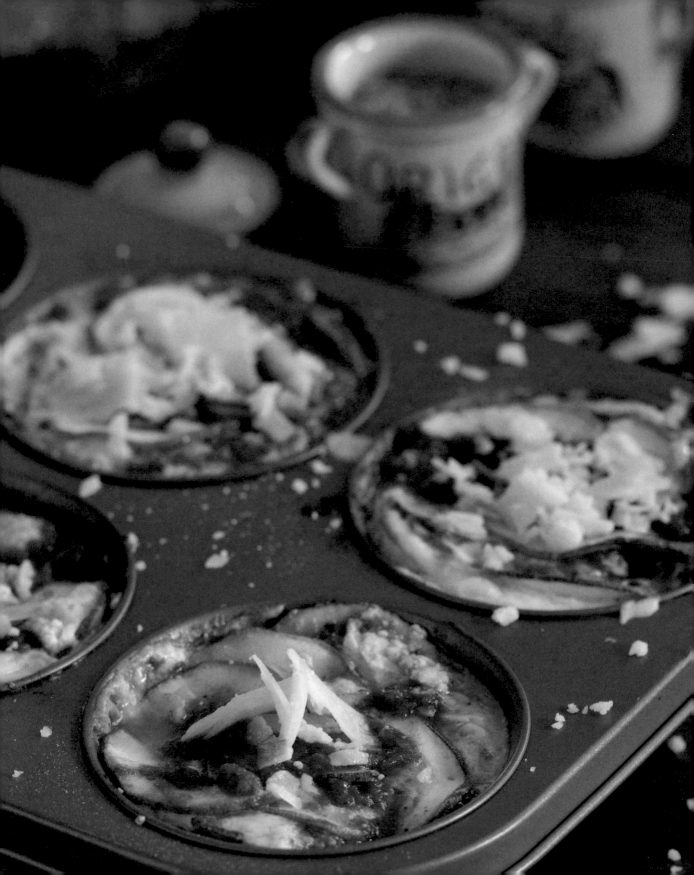

LASAGNA ROSETTES

HERE'S ANOTHER GREAT ALTERNATIVE to traditional lasagna. Because the zucchini will release moisture as it bakes, draining the ricotta is an essential step. Use your best olive oil for a flavorful finish.

MAKES 4 SERVINGS (2 ROSETTES PER SERVING)

Preheat the oven to 350°F. Brush 8 cups of a 12-cup muffin tin with olive oil.

Trim the ends of both zucchini and use a vegetable peeler to slice them into thin ribbons. Arrange equal portions of the ribbons in the 8 prepared muffin cups, reserving some for the top.

Remove excess moisture from the ricotta by placing it in the center of a piece of cheesecloth several layers thick. Draw up the ends and twist the cheesecloth over the sink to wring out the water.

In a large bowl, mix the drained ricotta, eggs, basil, and oregano. Season with the salt and pepper. Divide the mixture among the prepared muffin cups. Top each cup with 1 tablespoon of mozzarella and 1 tablespoon of tomato paste, followed by the remaining zucchini ribbons.

Bake for 15 minutes until set. Let cool for about 20 minutes before removing them from the muffin cups. Drizzle with the olive oil. Garnish with the Parmesan before serving.

CALORIES 385 | PROTEIN 24 G (24%) | CARBS 15 G (15%) | FAT 27 G (61%)
SAT FAT 10.9 G | FIBER 3 G

2 large zucchini

1 cup ricotta

6 eggs

½ teaspoon dried basil

½ teaspoon dried oregano

Salt and freshly ground black pepper

½ cup shredded mozzarella cheese

½ cup tomato paste

2 tablespoons olive oil

3 tablespoons grated Parmesan cheese

CHEESY SQUASH CASSEROLE

THIS IS AN IDEAL RECIPE TO ENJOY when your garden is overflowing with summer squash. Should yellow squash not be available, zucchini makes a perfect substitute.

MAKES 4 SERVINGS

1 onion, divided

3 eggs, lightly beaten

3 tablespoons mayonnaise

1 tablespoon garlic powder

2 pounds yellow squash, spiralized into noodles (about 6 cups)

1½ cups Cheddar cheese, divided

Salt and freshly ground black pepper

1 tablespoon olive oil

¼ cup grated Parmesan cheese

Preheat the oven to 400°F. Brush a 3-quart baking dish with olive oil.

Halve the onion from stem to root and finely chop one half. In a large bowl, mix the onion, the eggs, mayonnaise, and garlic powder, and stir until thoroughly combined. Add the squash and 1 cup of Cheddar. Season to taste with the salt and pepper. Mix with your hands until the squash is thoroughly coated. Transfer the mixture to the prepared dish and top with the remaining ½ cup Cheddar.

Slice the remaining half of the onion into very thin pieces and place into a smaller bowl. Drizzle the onion slices with olive oil and sprinkle with the Parmesan. Season to taste with salt and pepper. Toss to coat.

Scatter the onion mixture on top of the casserole. Bake, covered, for 30 minutes, until the squash is tender and the cheese is bubbling. Uncover and bake another 10 minutes until the top begins to brown. Let cool slightly before serving.

CALORIES 410 | PROTEIN 20 G (19%) | CARBS 12 G (11%) | FAT 33 G (70%)
SAT FAT 12.3 G | FIBER 3 G

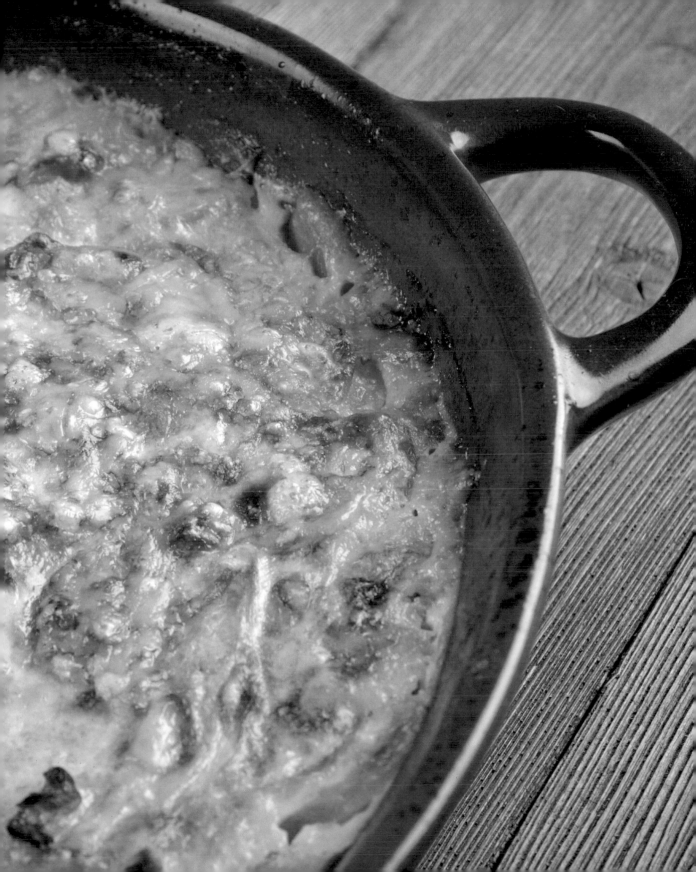

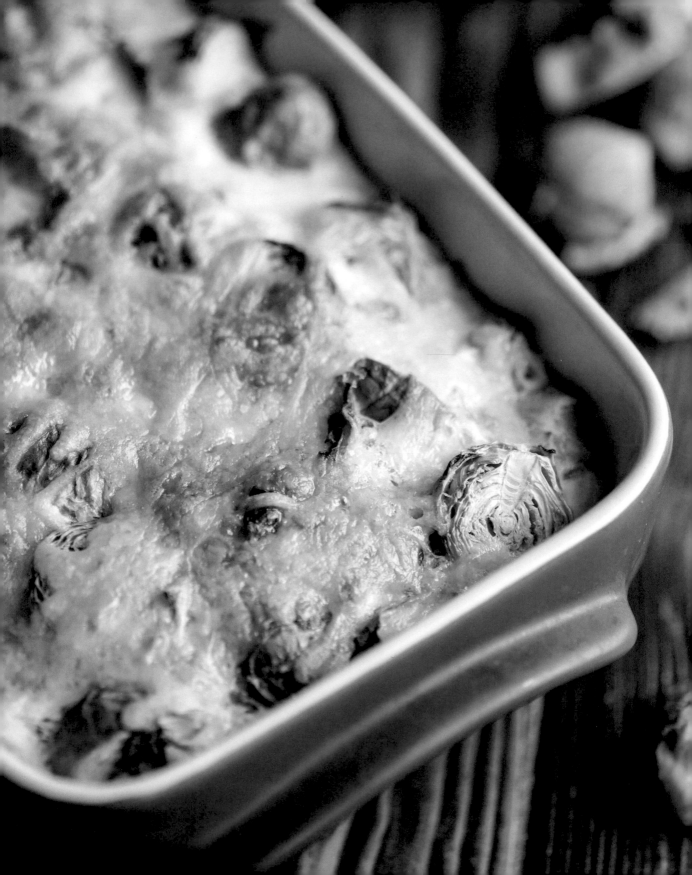

BETTER-WITHOUT-BACON BRUSSELS SPROUTS CASSEROLE

BRUSSELS SPROUTS PAIRED WITH BACON seems like a match made in heaven, and you can certainly add bacon to this recipe if you're so inclined. But with the addition of cream and rich Swiss cheeses, this dish tastes just fine with smoked almonds instead.

MAKES 8 SERVINGS

Preheat the oven to 400°F. Line a baking sheet with parchment paper. Brush a 9- x 13-inch baking dish with olive oil.

Place the brussels sprouts on the baking sheet and drizzle on the oil. Season to taste with the salt and pepper. Toss lightly to coat. Spread the brussels sprouts evenly on the sheet and bake for 20 minutes.

In a large bowl, combine the cream, eggs, cheeses, rosemary, garlic powder, and paprika and stir until thoroughly mixed.

Transfer the brussels sprouts to the baking dish and cover them with the cream mixture. Scatter the almonds on top. Reduce the oven temperature to 350°F. Bake for 20 to 30 minutes, until the cheese is bubbling and beginning to brown.

CALORIES 315 | PROTEIN 13 G (16%) | CARBS 11 G (13%) | FAT 26 G (71%)
SAT FAT 11.7 G | FIBER 4 G

1½ pounds brussels sprouts, cut in halves

2 tablespoons olive oil

Salt and freshly ground black pepper

1 cup heavy cream

2 eggs, lightly beaten

1 cup grated Jarlsburg cheese

½ cup grated Gruyere cheese

1½ teaspoons chopped fresh rosemary or ½ teaspoon dried

1 teaspoon garlic powder

1 teaspoon smoked paprika

½ cup smoked almonds, coarsely chopped

EASY CAULIFLOWER MAC & CHEESE

HERE'S A COMFORT FOOD CLASSIC that comes together conveniently if you rely on chopped frozen cauliflower. Of course, if you have a fresh large head on hand, that works fine too. You'll need about 6 cups of raw florets for this recipe.

MAKES 4 SERVINGS

2 pounds frozen cauliflower florets

¾ cup heavy cream

4 ounces cream cheese

Salt and freshly ground black pepper

2 cups shredded Cheddar cheese, divided

1 teaspoon Dijon mustard

1 teaspoon ground turmeric

½ teaspoon garlic powder

In a large pot, heat a cup of water over medium-high heat and add the cauliflower. Cook, covered, for about 10 minutes until the cauliflower is tender but not mushy.

In a small pot, warm the cream over medium heat until it begins to bubble. Add the cream cheese and stir the mixture until smooth. Season to taste with the salt and pepper. Add 1½ cups of the Cheddar and stir until smooth. Add the mustard, turmeric, and garlic powder, and taste to adjust seasonings.

Drain the cauliflower and transfer it to a large bowl. Cover it with the cheese sauce. Toss to coat. Scatter the remaining ½ cup of Cheddar on top, and serve once the cheese has melted.

CALORIES 480 | PROTEIN 19 G (16%) | CARBS 11 G (9%) | FAT 41 G (75%)
SAT FAT 22.4 G | FIBER 6 G

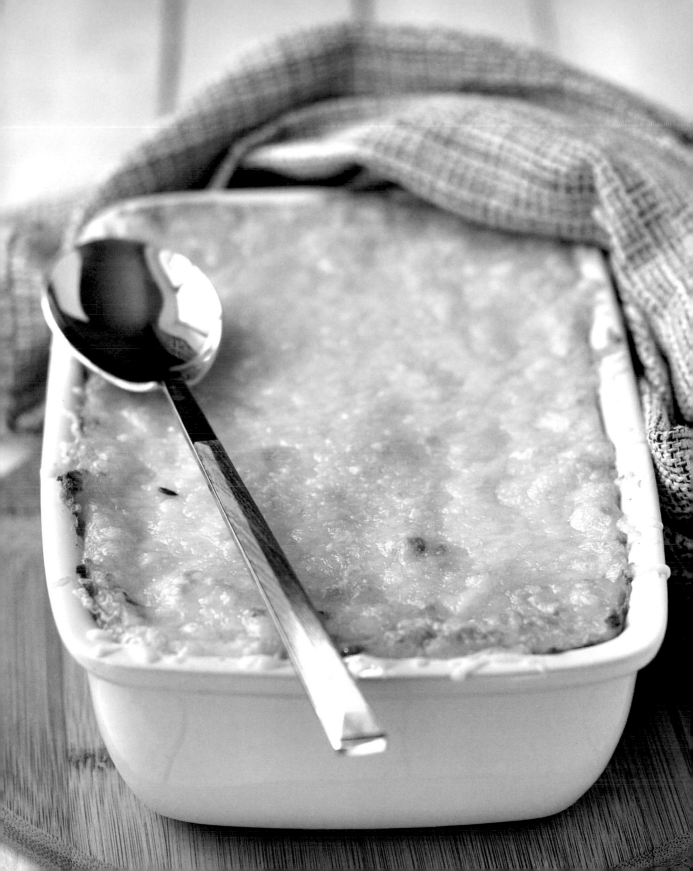

GARLICKY SHRIMP *over Tomatoes*

THIS POPULAR SPANISH DISH is traditionally served with a crusty bread to sop up the irresistible garlic sauce, but fresh tomatoes are keto-friendly and just as delicious. Use large shrimp if your budget allows.

MAKES 4 SERVINGS

1½ pounds shrimp, peeled and deveined

1 teaspoon smoked paprika

Salt and freshly ground black pepper

½ cup olive oil

10 large cloves garlic, minced

1 teaspoon red pepper flakes

Juice of 1 lemon

1 tablespoon chopped fresh parsley

2 large beefsteak tomatoes, sliced

Toss the shrimp with the paprika and season to taste with the salt and pepper. Set aside. In a large heavy skillet, warm the oil over medium heat. Add the garlic and red pepper flakes and cook for about 1 minute or until the garlic just begins to brown.

Raise to high heat and immediately add the shrimp and lemon juice. Cook, stirring occasionally, until the shrimp turn pink and curl, about 3 minutes.

Adjust seasonings and serve the shrimp on top of the tomato slices. Sprinkle with parsley just before serving.

CALORIES 400 | PROTEIN 25 G (25%) | CARBS 10 G (10%) | FAT 29 G (65%)
SAT FAT 4.2 G | FIBER 2 G

FISH TACOS
with Cashew-Avocado Crema

THESE FESTIVE TACOS are worthy of a party. While they contain more carbs than many recipes in this collection, they are well within a reasonable ketogenic diet range if you plan your day accordingly.

MAKES 4 SERVINGS

TO MAKE THE CREMA: Drain the cashews and combine with the lime juice, garlic, and salt in a blender; whirl, adding just enough water (if necessary) until the mixture reaches a thick, smooth consistency. Add the avocado and pulse again until smooth. Set aside.

TO MAKE THE TACOS: Place the fish in a shallow dish and sprinkle with the cumin, garlic powder, and cayenne (if using). Toss to coat. In a large skillet, warm the oil over medium heat, and add the fish. Cover and cook 5 to 7 minutes, shaking the skillet every few minutes, until the fish is no longer opaque and a fork slides easily through a thick piece. Remove from the heat and toss with the lime juice and cilantro. To assemble the tacos, top each lettuce leaf with equal portions of fish, pepper slices, onion, and crema.

CALORIES 465 | PROTEIN 28 G (23%) | CARBS 19 G (16%) | FAT 33 G (61%)
SAT FAT 5.5 G | FIBER 8 G

Cashew-Avocado Crema
½ cup cashews, soaked in 1 cup water 2 to 4 hours

Juice of 1½ limes

2 cloves garlic

¼ teaspoon salt

1 avocado, peeled

Fish Tacos
1 pound mild white fish, preferably snapper, cut into 1½-inch pieces

1 teaspoon ground cumin

1 teaspoon garlic powder

¼ teaspoon ground cayenne (optional)

3 tablespoons olive oil

Juice of ½ lime

½ bunch fresh cilantro, chopped

1 head Boston lettuce, washed and separated

1 bell pepper, sliced

½ small red onion, sliced

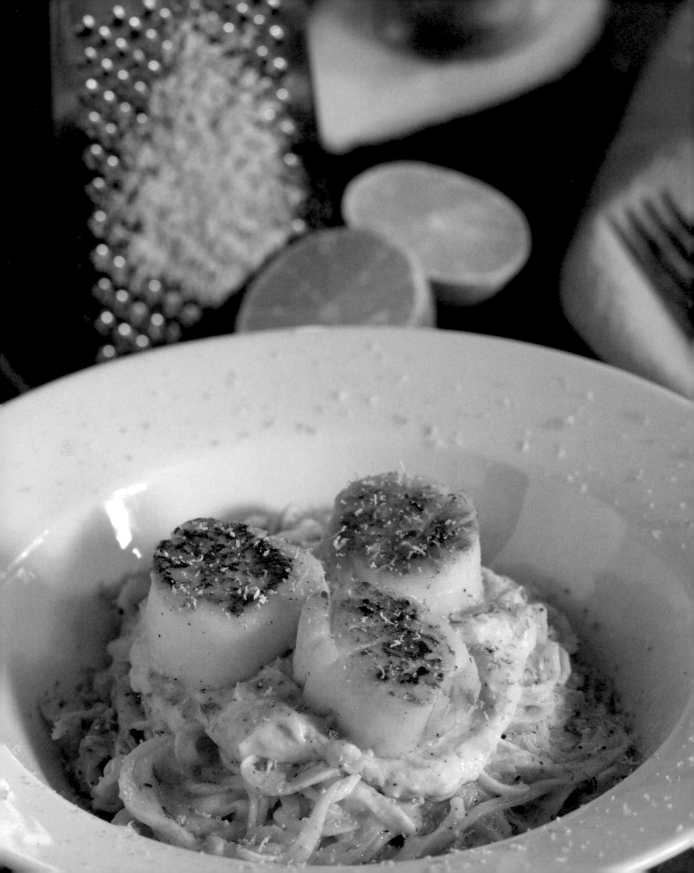

SCALLOPS WITH YELLOW SQUASH "NOODLES"
and Avocado-Lime Sauce

TIMING IS EVERYTHING when it comes to cooking the perfect scallop. While this dish comes together quickly, it's best to prepare the Avocado-Lime Sauce first so that you can plate your entire dish as soon as the scallops are done.

MAKES 4 SERVINGS

TO MAKE THE AVOCADO SAUCE: Place the avocado, oil, lime juice, and mayonnaise in a blender and whirl until smooth. Taste and add a dash of salt (if using).

TO MAKE THE SCALLOPS AND "NOODLES": In a large skillet, melt the butter over medium heat. Add the squash and garlic. Cook, stirring occasionally, for 3 minutes until the squash is tender. Season to taste with the salt and pepper. Remove the skillet from the heat while you prepare the scallops.

Use a paper towel to pat the scallops dry. Sprinkle with salt and pepper.

In a large skillet, heat the oil over high heat. Add the scallops, flat-side down, and cook for 2 to 3 minutes until the edges begin to brown. Flip and cook 1 minute longer until the scallops are firm. Serve the noodles topped with the avocado sauce and scallops. Scatter zest on top of each portion and add a squeeze of lime juice just before serving.

CALORIES 405 | PROTEIN 20 G (19%) | CARBS 15 G (14%) | FAT 31 G (67%)
SAT FAT 7.3 G | FIBER 4 G

Avocado-Lime Sauce
1 avocado, peeled

2 tablespoons olive oil

Juice of ½ lime

2 tablespoons mayonnaise

Salt (optional)

Scallops and "Noodles"
2 tablespoons butter

2 large yellow squash, trimmed and spiralized into thick noodles

2 cloves garlic, minced

Salt and freshly ground black pepper

2 tablespoons olive oil

12 jumbo sea scallops (about 1¼ pounds)

Zest of 1 lime

Juice of ½ lime

SALMON AND ASPARAGUS STIR-FRY

CHILI GARLIC SAUCE IS POPULAR in Asian cuisine and contains ground chile peppers, garlic, salt, and vinegar. If you enjoy spicy food, you'll likely find an unlimited number of uses for this remarkably full-bodied condiment. If you prefer more mild dishes, feel free to use less-assertive hot sauce in its place, or omit altogether.

MAKES 4 SERVINGS

1 pound skinless salmon fillet, cut into 1½-inch pieces

Salt and freshly ground pepper

2 tablespoons reduced-sodium soy sauce

1 tablespoon grated fresh ginger

1 tablespoon chili garlic sauce (optional)

2 tablespoons toasted sesame oil

1 pound asparagus, trimmed and cut into 1½-inch pieces (about 2 cups)

1 cup chopped cashews

Season the fish with salt and pepper. In a small bowl, whisk together the soy sauce, ginger, and chili garlic sauce (if using). Set aside.

In a large wok, heat the oil over medium-high heat. Add the salmon and cook for 2 to 3 minutes until it is firm and opaque. Transfer the fish to a plate.

Without wiping out the wok, add the asparagus and 2 tablespoons of water. Cover and let cook until the asparagus is bright green and tender, about 3 to 4 minutes. Pour the soy sauce mixture over the asparagus and cook, uncovered, about 1 minute longer. Return the salmon to the wok and toss gently to coat. Top the salmon with the cashews just before serving.

CALORIES 470 | PROTEIN 35 G (29%) | CARBS 16 G (13%) | FAT 31 G (58%)
SAT FAT 10.9 G | FIBER 3 G

BAKED SALMON *with Tapenade*

YOU MAY WISH TO SKIP THE SALT altogether in this dish; the olives pack plenty of salty flavor, which you may find sufficiently satisfying.

MAKES 4 SERVINGS

Preheat the oven to 400°F. Line a baking sheet with parchment paper.

In the work bowl of a food processor, combine the olives, parsley, olive oil, capers, lemon juice, and garlic and pulse until finely chopped.

Season the fish with the salt and pepper and arrange, skin-side down, on the baking sheet. Spread the olive mixture evenly over the top of the fish. Bake for 20 minutes or until the fish flakes easily with a fork. Serve on a bed of arugula.

CALORIES 420 | PROTEIN 42 G (40%) | CARBS 4 G (4%) | FAT 26 G (56%)
SAT FAT 4 G | FIBER 2 G

1 cup pitted Kalamata olives

¼ cup coarsely chopped fresh parsley

3 tablespoons olive oil

2 teaspoons capers

1 teaspoon fresh lemon juice

1 clove garlic

1½ pounds salmon fillets

Salt and freshly ground black pepper

4 cups arugula

SPICY TUNA PATTIES

TUNA PATTIES ARE A CLASSIC COMFORT FOOD, but here they enjoy a new twist with the addition of a spicy mayo topping in place of a traditional tartar sauce.

MAKES 4 SERVINGS

3 cans (5-ounce) albacore tuna in water, drained

¼ yellow onion, diced

½ cup mayonnaise, divided

1 egg, lightly beaten

¼ cup almond flour

1 jalapeño pepper, diced

Juice of ½ lemon

Salt and freshly ground black pepper

3 tablespoons olive oil

2 tablespoons chipotle pepper sauce

In a large bowl, mix the tuna, onion, cup mayonnaise, egg, almond flour, jalapeño, and lemon juice until thoroughly combined. Season to taste with the salt and pepper. Divide the mixture into 8 equal portions and form into patties.

In a large skillet, warm the oil over medium-high heat and cook the patties 3 minutes per side until golden brown and crisp on the outside. While the patties cook, whisk together the remaining ¼ cup of mayonnaise and pepper sauce to serve on top.

CALORIES 515 | PROTEIN 34 G (26%) | CARBS 5 G (4%) | FAT 40 G (70%)
SAT FAT 6.3 G | FIBER 1.5 G

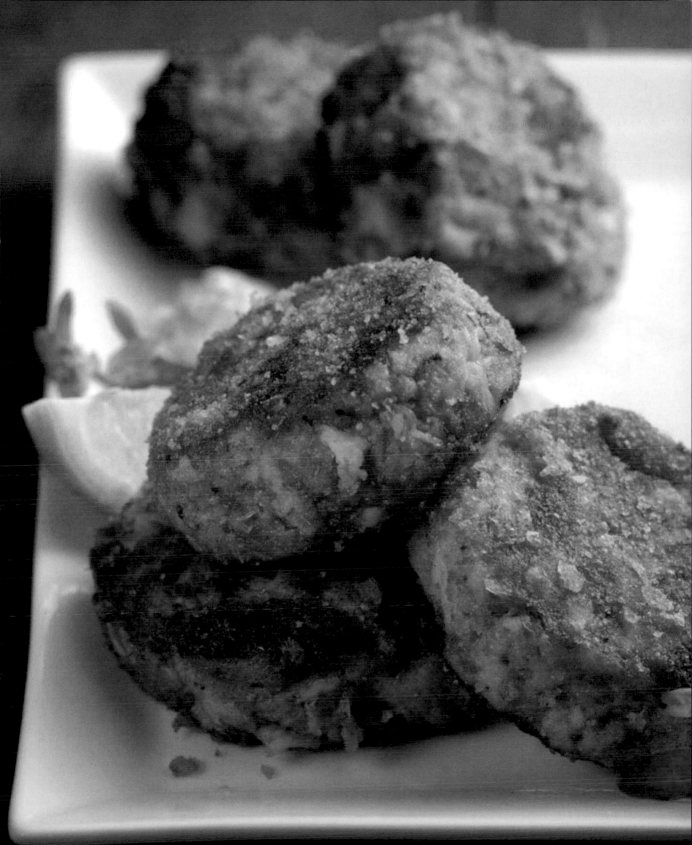

BUTTERY ROAST COD
with Crunchy Almond Topping

SERVE THIS DISH alongside cooked green beans if you like. A half cup serving contains 5 grams of carbohydrates.

MAKES 4 SERVINGS

1 pound cod fillets

Salt and freshly ground black pepper

¼ cup butter, melted

2 tablespoons fresh lemon juice

1 teaspoon lemon zest

¼ cup toasted slivered almonds

1 scallion, thinly sliced

Preheat the oven to 400°F. Season the fish with salt and pepper and arrange in an 8- x 8-inch baking dish.

In a small bowl, whisk the butter, lemon juice, and lemon zest. Pour the sauce over the fish and bake it for 20 minutes until it is opaque and flakes easily with a fork.

Top with the almonds and scallion slices before serving.

CALORIES 285 | PROTEIN 25 G (35%) | CARBS 3 G (4%) | FAT 19 G (61%)
SAT FAT 8.4 G | FIBER 1 G

COCONUT CURRY COD
with Cauliflower "Rice"

COD IS A FLAVOR-NEUTRAL FISH that serves as an excellent backdrop for the flavorful curry sauce in this dish. Each serving of cauliflower "rice" provides 9 grams of carbohydrates and 5 grams of fiber, which is good information to have if you choose to serve it as a side for another dish.

MAKES 4 SERVINGS

Preheat the oven to 400°F. Season the fish with salt and pepper and arrange in an 8- x 8-inch baking dish.

Use a box grater or a food processor with the grater attachment to chop the cauliflower into rice-size pieces, leaving any large, tough stems behind. Transfer the cauliflower to a clean towel or paper towel and press to remove excess moisture. Set aside.

In a small bowl, whisk together the coconut milk, ginger, and curry paste until smooth. (Microwave the mixture for a minute, if necessary, to make ingredients easier to combine.) Pour the sauce over the fish and bake for 20 minutes, until it is opaque and flakes easily with a fork.

In a large skillet, heat the oil over medium heat. Cook the cauliflower, covered, for 5 to 8 minutes, until tender. Season to taste with the salt and pepper.

Serve the fish and sauce over the "rice." Top with cilantro (if using) just before serving.

CALORIES 430 | PROTEIN 29 G (26%) | CARBS 12 G (11%) | FAT 31 G (63%)
SAT FAT 18.3 G | FIBER 5 G

1 pound cod fillets

Salt and freshly ground black pepper

1 large head cauliflower florets

1½ cups coconut milk

2 teaspoons grated fresh ginger

2 teaspoons green curry paste

1 tablespoon olive oil

2 tablespoons chopped fresh cilantro (optional)

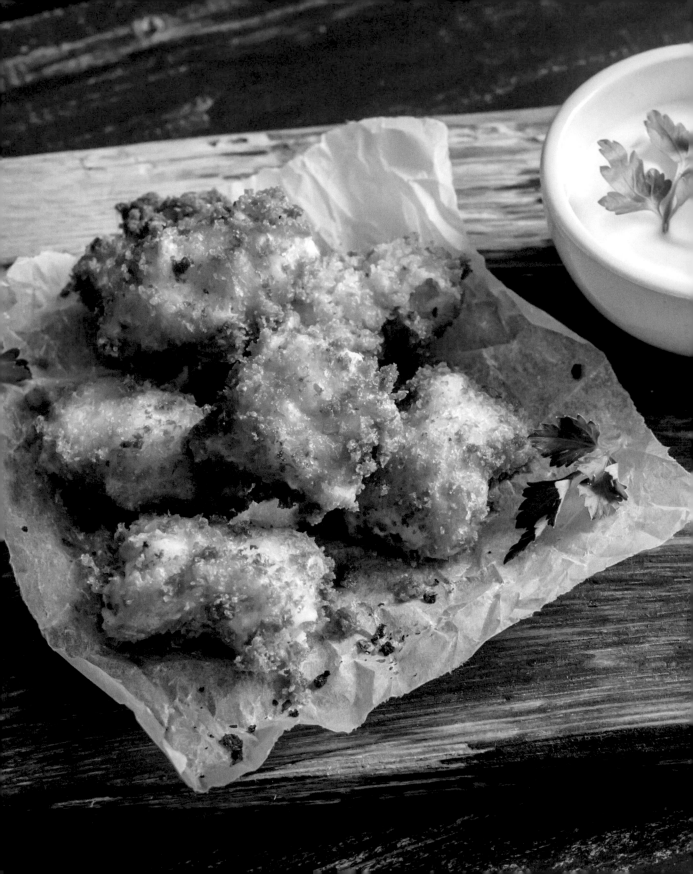

OVEN "FRIED" CATFISH
with Spicy Dipping Sauce

GRATED PARMESAN WORKS PERFECTLY as a lower-carb breading. You won't even miss the breadcrumbs! Serve with a side of slaw (no sugar added, of course).

MAKES 4 SERVINGS

Preheat the oven to 400°F. Line a baking sheet with parchment paper.

In a gallon-size resealable plastic bag, combine the Parmesan, flaxseed, almond flour, and Old Bay seasoning and shake lightly until thoroughly mixed. In a shallow bowl, lightly beat the egg with a tablespoon of water.

Working in batches, dip the fish pieces in the egg wash and then drop them into the bag with the seasoning mixture. Shake gently until the fish pieces are thoroughly coated, then arrange them on the baking sheet. Press any remaining coating crumbs into the fish. Bake for 10 minutes or until a fork slips easily through the thickest piece of fish.

While the fish is baking, whisk together the mayonnaise, hot sauce, and lemon juice. Serve the sauce with the fish for dipping.

CALORIES 570 | PROTEIN 37 G (26%) | CARBS 6 G (4%) | FAT 44 G (70%)
SAT FAT 9.7 G | FIBER 3 G

⅓ cup + 1 tablespoon grated Parmesan cheese

¼ cup ground flaxseed

2 tablespoons almond flour

1 tablespoon Old Bay seasoning

1 egg

1½ pounds catfish, cut into 1½-inch pieces

⅓ cup mayonnaise

1 tablespoon hot sauce

1 teaspoon fresh lemon juice

ROAST HALIBUT
with Garlic Sauce and Greens

HERE'S A HANDY TIP that will make your garlic chopping routine much easier. Sprinkle a little salt on the garlic beforehand, and you'll notice far less of it sticking to the sides of your knife while you chop.

MAKES 4 SERVINGS

1½ pounds halibut fillet

Salt and freshly ground black pepper

⅓ cup mayonnaise

3 cloves garlic, finely minced

3 tablespoons olive oil, divided

1 teaspoon lemon zest

1½ pounds Swiss chard, coarsely chopped

2 tablespoons fresh lemon juice

Preheat the oven to 400°F. Season the fish with salt and pepper and arrange in an 8- x 8-inch baking dish.

In a small bowl, whisk together the mayonnaise, garlic, 2 tablespoons of the oil, and the zest. Spread the mixture evenly over the fish and bake for 20 minutes until it is opaque and flakes easily with a fork.

In a large skillet, warm the remaining tablespoon of oil over medium-high heat. Add the chard and 2 tablespoons of water and cook, covered, stirring occasionally, for 5 to 7 minutes until the greens are tender. Drizzle on the lemon juice and season to taste with the salt and pepper.

Arrange the fish on a bed of greens. Drizzle any remaining sauce over the fish before serving.

CALORIES 410 | PROTEIN 35 G (34%) | CARBS 8 G (7 %) | FAT 27 G (59%)
SAT FAT 4 G | FIBER 3 G

BUFFALO CHICKEN TENDERS

ONE OF THE BENEFITS OF A KETOGENIC weight loss plan is that you don't have to forego flavor when it comes to dishes that traditionally rely on a bit of butter, which in this particular recipe is used to temper the vinegary spice of the hot sauce. An added bonus: Regular blue cheese dressing is just fine too!

MAKES 4 SERVINGS

Preheat the oven to 350°F. Line a baking sheet with parchment paper.

Season the chicken tenders with the salt and freshly ground black pepper. In a gallon-size resealable plastic bag, add the almond flour and season to taste with the salt and pepper. In a small shallow bowl, beat the egg and heavy cream.

Working with a few pieces at a time, dip the chicken tenders into the egg wash and then drop them into the bag with the flour. Seal the bag, shake to coat, and then arrange the tenders on the baking sheet. Repeat with the remaining ingredients. Bake for 15 to 20 minutes, flipping halfway through, until a thermometer inserted into the center of the tenders reaches 165°F.

Stir together the hot sauce and butter. Pour the hot sauce mixture over the tenders before serving with the blue cheese dressing and celery.

CALORIES 610 | PROTEIN 40 G (26%) | CARBS 9 G (6%) | FAT 46 G (68%)
SAT FAT 12.6 G | FIBER 4 G

1¼ pounds chicken tenders

Salt and freshly ground black pepper

1 cup almond flour

1 egg

1 tablespoon heavy cream

¼ cup hot sauce

¼ cup butter, melted

½ cup blue cheese dressing

1 bunch celery, trimmed and cut into sticks

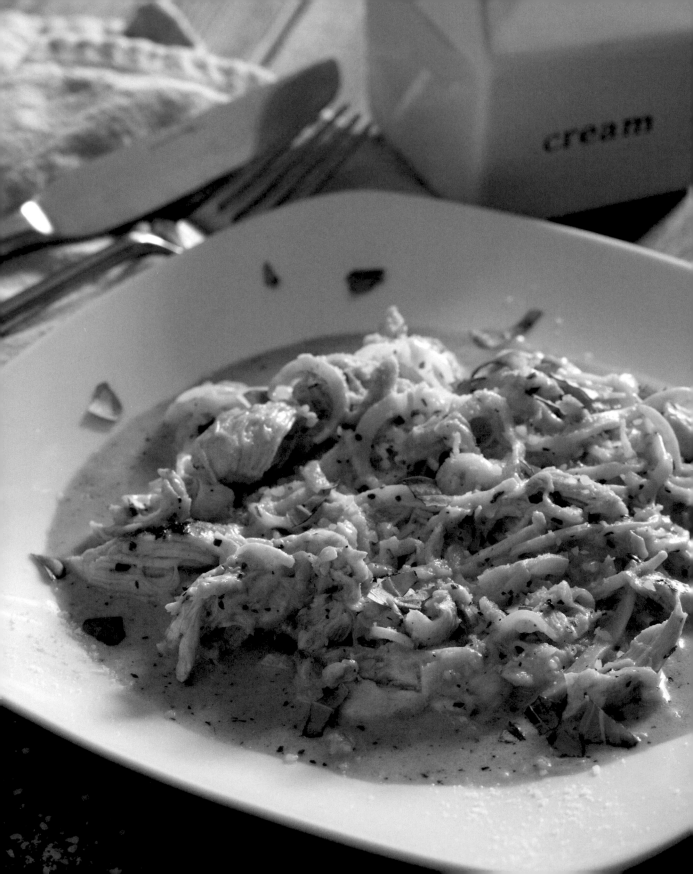

CHICKEN SQUASH ALFREDO

AN ADDED BONUS of using your own spiralized veggie noodles instead of regular pasta: No need to wait for a pot of water to boil! Once you've prepped your ingredients, this dish comes together in about 10 minutes flat.

MAKES 4 SERVINGS

In a large heavy skillet, melt the butter over medium-high heat. Add the garlic and cook, stirring, for 30 seconds until fragrant. Add the heavy cream and simmer for 3 minutes to allow flavors to combine. Add the Parmesan a few spoonfuls at a time, stirring after each addition, until melted.

Add the squash and chicken. Cook, stirring occasionally, for about 5 minutes until noodles are tender but not mushy and the chicken is heated through. Season to taste with the salt and pepper. Top with the basil just before serving.

CALORIES 290 | PROTEIN 7 G (9%) | CARBS 9 G (12%) | FAT 26 G (79%)
SAT FAT 16.1 G | FIBER 2 G

¼ cup butter

4 cloves garlic, minced

½ cup heavy cream

½ cup grated Parmesan cheese

2 large yellow squash, trimmed and spiralized into noodles

2 cups cooked shredded chicken

Salt and freshly ground black pepper

¼ cup chopped fresh basil

CHICKEN PARMESAN

HERE'S AN ITALIAN CLASSIC that proves you really don't need bread crumbs, or pasta for that matter, to enjoy all the flavors of this delicious dish. If you don't have fresh mozzarella handy, regular shredded mozzarella will do just fine.

MAKES 4 SERVINGS

2 boneless, skinless chicken breasts (about ¾ pound)

Salt and freshly ground black pepper

1 egg

½ cup grated Parmesan cheese

1 teaspoon garlic powder

1 teaspoon dried oregano

3 tablespoon olive oil

2 cloves garlic, minced

2 large zucchini (about 1½ pounds), trimmed and spiralized into noodles

1½ cups no-sugar-added marinara sauce, divided

2 ounces fresh mozzarella cheese, sliced

¼ cup fresh chopped basil

Preheat the oven to 400°F. Line a baking sheet with parchment paper.

Put the chicken breasts on a flat work surface. Placing the palm of your hand flat on top of one breast and holding your knife parallel to the work surface, carefully slice the chicken horizontally to make 2 cutlets. Repeat with the remaining chicken breast. Season the chicken with the salt and pepper. Set aside.

In a shallow bowl, lightly beat the egg with a tablespoon of water. In another shallow bowl, add the Parmesan, garlic powder, and oregano. Stir until thoroughly combined. Dip one chicken cutlet into the egg wash and then the Parmesan mixture, pressing it onto the chicken to form a crust. Place the chicken on the baking sheet. Repeat with the remaining cutlets. Bake for 15 minutes.

In a large skillet, heat the oil over medium-high heat. Add the garlic and cook, stirring, for about 30 seconds until fragrant. Add the zucchini noodles and cook for 2 minutes, tossing frequently, until they are tender. Season to taste with the salt and pepper. Add 1 cup of the marinara and toss to coat. Cook 1 minute longer until marinara is heated through. Transfer the noodles to a serving dish and cover them lightly with foil to keep warm.

Remove the chicken from the oven. Arrange the mozzarella evenly on each chicken breast, followed by 2 tablespoons of marinara. Return the chicken to the oven and continue baking for another 5 minutes, or until the mozzarella is melted and the temperature in the thickest part of the chicken registers 165°F. Remove the chicken from the oven and arrange each piece on the noodles. Garnish with the basil just before serving.

CALORIES 350 | PROTEIN 29 G (32%) | CARBS 14 G (16%) | FAT 21 G (52%)
SAT FAT 6 G | FIBER 4 G

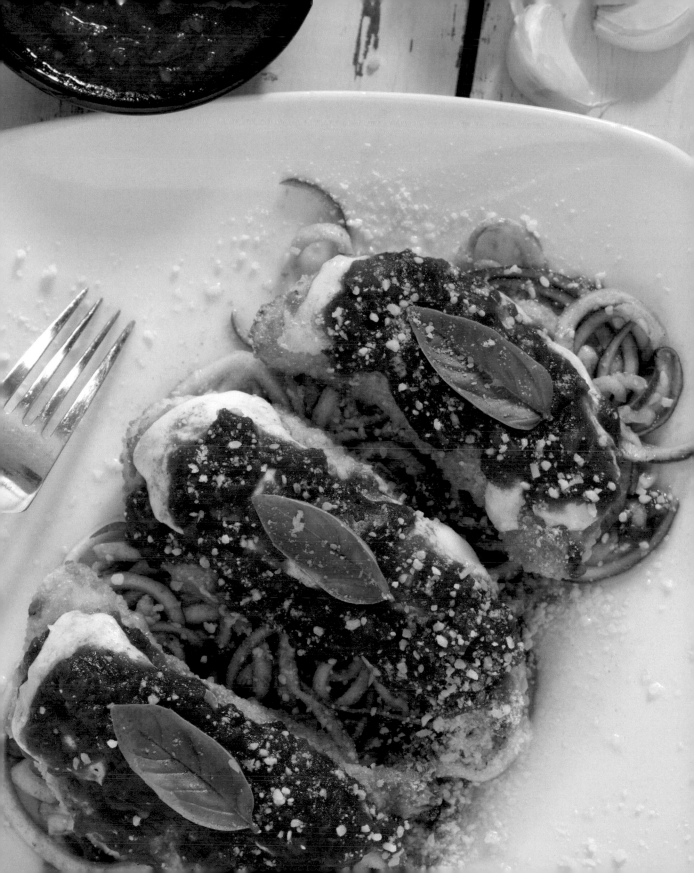

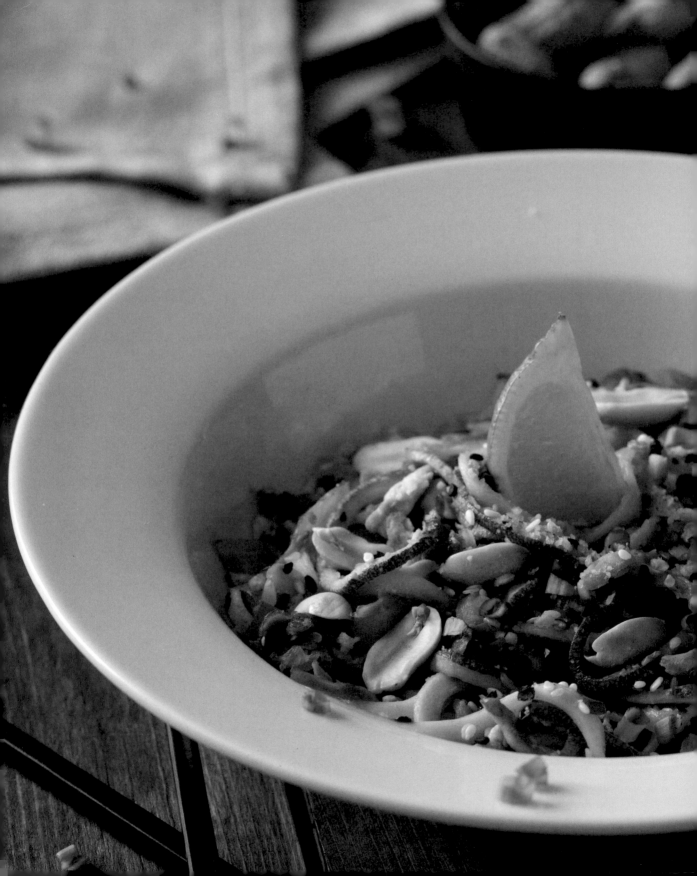

CHICKEN PAD THAI

YOU SKIP A FAIR AMOUNT OF CARBS when you opt for these zucchini noodles in place of the traditional rice noodles. The best part: All the flavors will make you forget that you're enjoying a low-carb feast. Omit the chili garlic paste if you're not a fan of spicy foods.

MAKES 4 SERVINGS

Slice half the lime into wedges. Squeeze the juice from the other half into a small bowl. Add the soy sauce and chili garlic paste (if using). Set aside.

In a wok, heat the oil over high heat. Add the onion, ginger, and garlic. Cook, stirring frequently, for 1 minute until the onion begins to soften. Add the chicken. Season to taste with the salt and pepper. Cook, stirring frequently, for 5 minutes until the chicken is cooked through. Transfer the chicken to a bowl and return the wok to the heat.

Add the eggs to the wok and cook, stirring occasionally, for 1 to 2 minutes until scrambled. Add the zucchini noodles and cook 2 minutes longer until they are tender. Pour the reserved soy mixture over the noodles along with the chicken and peanuts. Cook 1 minute longer, tossing frequently, to combine. Serve garnished with a lime wedge.

CALORIES 375 | PROTEIN 33 G (33%) | CARBS 14 G (14%) | FAT 23 G (53%)
SAT FAT 4 G | FIBER 4 G

1 lime

2 tablespoons reduced-sodium soy sauce

1 tablespoon chili garlic paste (optional)

1 tablespoon toasted sesame oil

½ onion, chopped

1 tablespoon grated fresh ginger

4 cloves garlic, minced

1 pound boneless, skinless chicken thighs, chopped

Salt and freshly ground black pepper

2 eggs, lightly beaten

2 large zucchini (about 1½ pounds), trimmed and spiralized into noodles

½ cup chopped peanuts

SPICY GRILLED CHICKEN
with Peanut Sauce

IF YOU WANT EXTRA ACCOMPANIMENTS, serve with a salad of thinly sliced cucumbers and radishes on a bed of lettuce. Alternately, keep the lettuce leaves whole, wrap them around the chicken alongside the other vegetables and garnishes, and use the peanut sauce for dipping.

MAKES 4 SERVINGS

⅓ cup reduced-sodium soy sauce

2 tablespoons Swerve or another zero-carb granulated sweetener

2 tablespoons olive oil

1 teaspoon chili garlic paste

Zest and juice of ½ lime

1½ pounds boneless, skinless chicken thighs, cut into 1-inch pieces

¼ cup chopped peanuts

¼ cup chopped fresh cilantro (for garnish)

Peanut Sauce

½ cup smooth peanut butter

4 to 5 tablespoons warm water

1 tablespoon reduced-sodium soy sauce

1 teaspoon chili garlic paste

Juice of ½ lime

In a resealable plastic bag, combine the soy sauce, sweetener, olive oil, chili garlic paste, zest, and lime juice. Add the chicken thighs and seal. Refrigerate for at least 2 hours or up to overnight.

Preheat a broiler or grill. Thread the chicken pieces onto metal skewers (if using bamboo skewers, soak them for at least 30 minutes beforehand). Grill or broil the chicken for 10 minutes, turning occasionally, until cooked through and temperature in the thickest part registers 165°F.

TO PREPARE THE PEANUT SAUCE: Combine the peanut butter, water, soy sauce, chili garlic paste, and lime juice in a blender and whirl until smooth.

CALORIES 510 | PROTEIN 46 G (35%) | CARBS 11 G (8%) | FAT 33 G (57%)
SAT FAT 6.3 G | FIBER 3 G

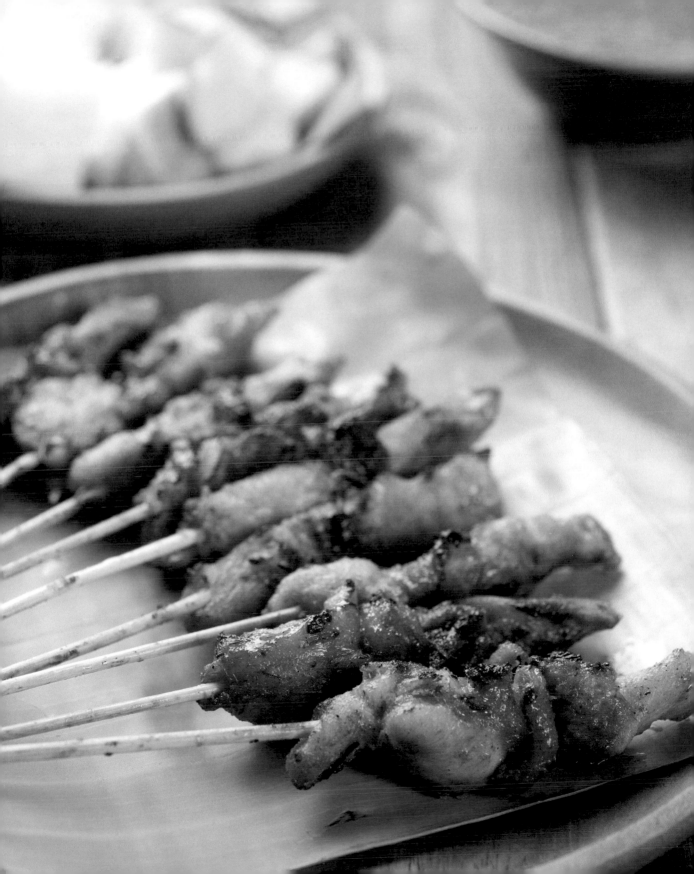

CHEESY CHICKEN-RELLENO CASSEROLE

HERE'S A RECIPE THAT COMES TOGETHER QUICKLY and is a great way to use up any leftover chicken you might have on hand. For a vegetarian version, simply omit the chicken.

MAKES 8 SERVINGS

2 cans (4.5-ounce) chopped green chiles, drained

2 cups shredded pepper jack cheese

1 cup cooked, shredded chicken

3 eggs

¾ cup heavy cream

Salt and freshly ground black pepper

1 cup shredded Cheddar cheese

2 scallions, thinly sliced (optional)

Preheat the oven to 350°F. Brush an 8- x 8-inch baking dish with olive oil.

Arrange half the chiles in the bottom of the dish, followed by alternating layers of the pepper jack cheese and chicken. Top with the remaining chiles.

In a small bowl, whisk together the eggs and cream until thoroughly combined. Season with the salt and pepper. Pour the egg mixture over the layered ingredients. Scatter the Cheddar on top.

Bake for 35 minutes until cooked through and the top is beginning to brown. Let cool for 10 minutes before slicing. Top with the scallion slices (if using).

CALORIES 510 | PROTEIN 35 G (27%) | CARBS 5 G (4%) | FAT 40 G (69%)
SAT FAT 23.3 G | FIBER 1 G

SLOW-COOKER CHICKEN CURRY
with Cauliflower "Rice"

CRAVING A SPICY BITE of Indian food? You can put together this easy curry in the morning and come home to a kitchen filled with delightful aromas.

MAKES 8 SERVINGS

Place the bell pepper, onion, and garlic in a slow cooker. Season the chicken with the salt and pepper and arrange on top of the vegetables. Whisk the coconut milk, broth, curry powder, and ginger until thoroughly combined. Pour over the chicken. Cover and cook on HIGH for 6 hours or LOW for 10 hours. In the last hour of cooking time, remove the chicken and pull the bones from the thighs. Return the chicken to the slow cooker and add the eggplant.

To prepare the cauliflower rice, use a box grater or a food processor with the grater attachment to chop the cauliflower into rice-size pieces, leaving any large, tough stems behind. Transfer the cauliflower to a clean towel or paper towel and press to remove excess moisture.

In a large skillet, heat the oil over medium heat. Cook the cauliflower, covered, for 5 to 8 minutes, until tender. Season to taste with the salt and pepper. Serve the curry over the "rice." Scatter the cilantro on top of each portion just before serving.

CALORIES 500 | PROTEIN 44 G (34%) | CARBS 15 G (12%) | FAT 31 G (54%)
SAT FAT 20.7 G | FIBER 6 G

1 red bell pepper, sliced

½ onion, chopped

6 cloves garlic, chopped

8 skinless chicken thighs (about 3½ pounds)

Salt and freshly ground black pepper

2 cans (13.5-ounce) coconut milk

⅓ cup reduced-sodium chicken broth

¼ cup curry powder

1 tablespoon grated fresh ginger

1 eggplant, peeled and chopped

1 large head cauliflower florets

1 tablespoon olive oil

½ cup chopped fresh cilantro

BROCCOLI-CHEDDAR CHICKEN CASSEROLE

LOOKING FOR A GOOD WAY to use those leftover chicken breasts in your fridge? Look no further. This comfort food classic feeds a crowd and is easy to assemble in minutes.

MAKES 6 SERVINGS

3 cups chopped cooked boneless, skinless chicken breast

2 cups chopped frozen broccoli

½ cup sour cream

½ cup heavy cream

2 tablespoons olive oil

½ teaspoon paprika

Salt and freshly ground black pepper

1 cup Cheddar cheese

½ cup crushed pork rinds

Preheat the oven to 400°F. Brush a 9- x 13-inch baking dish with olive oil.

In a large bowl, mix the chicken breast, broccoli, sour cream, heavy cream, olive oil, and paprika until thoroughly combined. Season with the salt and pepper. Transfer the chicken mixture to the prepared baking dish, spreading it evenly to the edges. Scatter the Cheddar and pork rinds on top.

Bake for 25 to 30 minutes until the top is browned and the cheese is bubbling. Let stand to cool slightly before serving.

CALORIES 365 | PROTEIN 34 G (37%) | CARBS 5 G (6%) | FAT 23 G (57%)
SAT FAT 10.4 G | FIBER 2 G

ZESTY TURKEY BURGERS

IF YOU'RE CRAVING a big juicy burger, turkey can satisfy. These simple burgers pack a big flavor punch.

MAKES 4 SERVINGS

In a large bowl, mix the turkey, onion, parsley, egg, Dijon, hot sauce, and garlic powder until thoroughly combined. Shape the mixture into 4 patties.

In a large skillet, warm the oil over medium-high heat. Fry the patties, 4 minutes per side, until cooked through and a thermometer inserted into the center of a patty registers 165°F. Transfer the patties to a plate and let rest for 5 minutes. To serve, place each patty in the center of a lettuce leaf and top with the avocado and tomato slices.

CALORIES 315 | PROTEIN 22 G (27%) | CARBS 9 G (11%) | FAT 22 G (62%)
SAT FAT 5.1 G | FIBER 4 G

1¼ pounds lean ground turkey

½ cup finely chopped onion

¼ cup chopped fresh parsley

1 egg

1 tablespoon Dijon mustard

1 tablespoon hot sauce

1 teaspoon garlic powder

2 teaspoons olive oil

4 large lettuce leaves

1 avocado, peeled and sliced

1 tomato, sliced

MEDITERRANEAN TURKEY MEATBALLS *with Lemon-Garlic Sauce*

THE BRIGHT FLAVORS OF LEMON AND GARLIC make these meatballs stand out. And because you're following a ketogenic weight loss plan, it's best to use full-fat yogurt. For an easy low-carb side, pair these meatballs with a cucumber salad topped with chopped Kalamata olives.

MAKES 4 SERVINGS

1¼ pounds lean ground turkey

¼ cup almond flour

1 egg

2 tablespoons chopped fresh dill or 2 teaspoons dried

½ teaspoon garlic powder

¼ teaspoon paprika

Salt and freshly ground black pepper

Lemon-Garlic Sauce

½ cup plain yogurt

¼ cup crumbled feta cheese

1 tablespoon chopped fresh dill or 1 teaspoon dried

1 tablespoon fresh lemon juice

1 tablespoon olive oil

1 clove garlic, minced

Preheat the oven to 375°F. Line a baking sheet with parchment paper.

In a large bowl, mix the turkey, almond flour, egg, dill, garlic powder, and paprika until thoroughly combined. Season with the salt and pepper. Roll 2 tablespoons of the turkey mixture into a ball and place it on the baking sheet. Repeat with the remaining mixture.

Bake for 20 minutes until the meatballs are cooked through and a thermometer inserted into the center of a meatball registers 165°F. Top with the lemon-garlic sauce just before serving.

TO PREPARE THE LEMON-GARLIC SAUCE: Combine the yogurt, feta, dill, lemon juice, olive oil, and garlic in a blender and whirl until smooth.

CALORIES 400 | PROTEIN 30 G (29%) | CARBS 5 G (5%) | FAT 30 G (66%) SAT FAT 8.1 G | FIBER 1 G

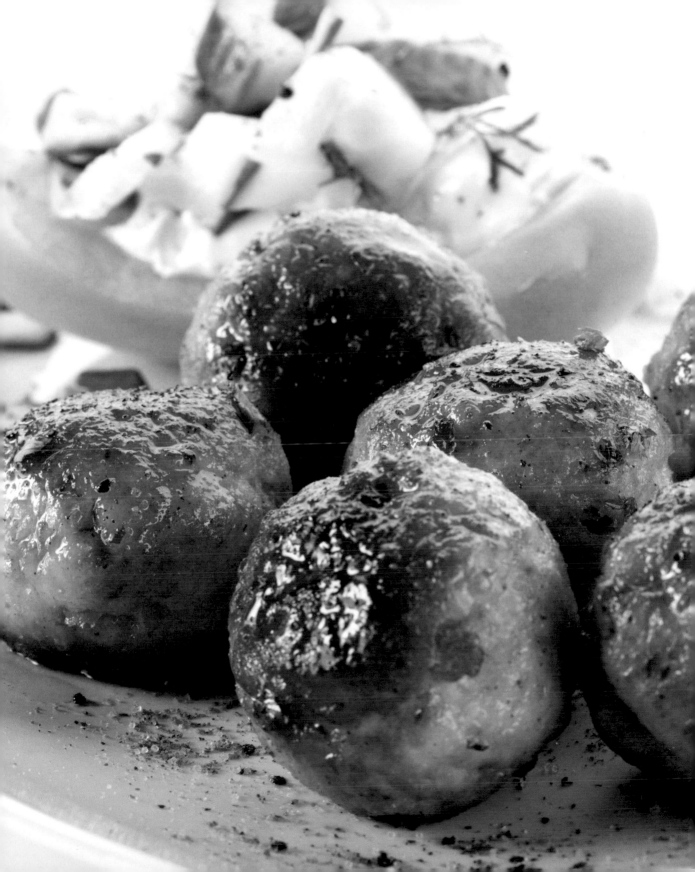

BEEF LO MEIN *with Shirataki Noodles*

SHIRATAKI NOODLES ARE ASIAN NOODLES made from a type of indigestible fiber, so often manufacturers can say that they are a zero-carb food. Look for them packaged in liquid and refrigerated in the produce section of your grocery store. If you prefer a different protein, replace the beef with chicken, pork, or shrimp.

MAKES 4 SERVINGS

2 bags (8-ounce) shirataki spaghetti noodles

2 tablespoons toasted sesame oil, divided

1 pound thinly sliced beef sirloin

2 tablespoons reduced-sodium soy sauce, divided

2 tablespoons smooth peanut butter

1 tablespoon grated fresh ginger

2 cloves garlic, minced

½ pound brown mushrooms, stemmed and sliced

½ red bell pepper, thinly sliced

½ onion, thinly sliced

2 cups shredded cabbage

1½ teaspoons chili garlic paste (optional)

3 scallions, thinly sliced

Drain the shirataki noodles in a colander and rinse well for a minute or 2 under running water. Cut the noodles into smaller pieces if they are exceedingly long. Set them aside.

In a wok or large skillet, heat 1 tablespoon of the oil over high heat. Cook the beef for 2 to 3 minutes, stirring frequently, until cooked through. Add 1 tablespoon of soy sauce and the peanut butter. Toss until the peanut butter has melted and coated the beef. Transfer the beef to a plate, making sure to scrape any sauce onto the plate as well. Carefully wipe out the wok with a paper towel and return the wok to the heat.

Warm the remaining tablespoon of oil. Add the ginger and garlic and cook for a minute until fragrant. Add the mushrooms, bell pepper, and onion and cook for 2 minutes longer until the vegetables begin to soften. Add the cabbage and remaining tablespoon of soy sauce. Cook, tossing occasionally, 1 minute longer until the vegetables are tender. Add the reserved noodles, beef (including any sauce on the plate), and chili garlic paste (if using). Cook, tossing occasionally, until ingredients are thoroughly combined and warmed through. Scatter the scallion slices on top of each serving.

CALORIES 385 | PROTEIN 28 G (28%) | CARBS 15 G (15% | FAT 25 G (57%)
SAT FAT 7.1 G | FIBER 5 G

SPICY BEEF *in Lettuce Cups*

HERE'S A GREAT WAY to use up any leftover cauliflower "rice" you might have on hand. With only 6 carbs per cup (and 2 grams of fiber), you'll be fine if you have a little more than the amount called for.

MAKES 4 SERVINGS

In a wok or large skillet, warm the oil over medium-high heat. Add the beef, breaking up the meat with the side of a spoon as it cooks, 5 to 7 minutes or until browned. Add the onion, ginger, fish sauce, and curry paste. Cook, stirring occasionally, 1 to 2 minutes longer until the onions soften and the ingredients are thoroughly combined. Remove from the heat.

Stir in the water chestnuts, cauliflower rice, lime juice, basil, and cilantro. Toss until the ingredients are thoroughly combined and heated through. Divide the mixture among the butter lettuce leaves and top with the peanuts before serving.

CALORIES 435 | PROTEIN 29 G (26%) | CARBS 17 G (15%) | FAT 30 G (59%)
SAT FAT 8.2 G | FIBER 5 G

1 tablespoon olive oil

1 pound lean ground beef

½ onion, chopped

1 tablespoon grated fresh ginger

2 teaspoons fish sauce

2 teaspoons red curry paste

1 can (8-ounce) sliced water chestnuts, drained and coarsely chopped

1 cup cauliflower rice

Juice of ½ lime

¼ cup chopped fresh basil

¼ cup chopped fresh cilantro

2 heads butter lettuce, separated into whole leaves

½ cup chopped peanuts

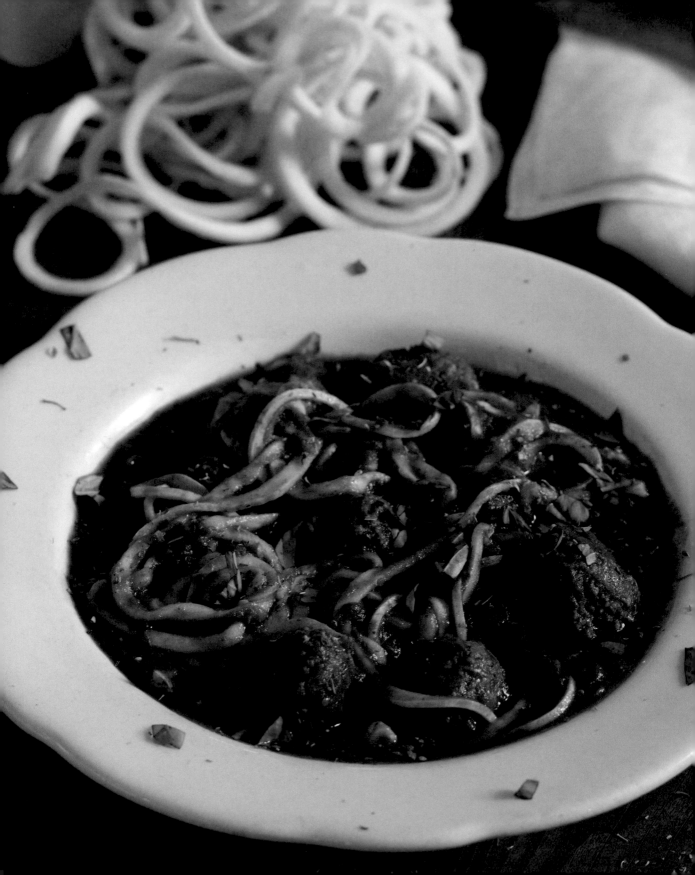

SPAGHETTI AND MEATBALLS MARINARA

IF YOU WANT TO PERSUADE YOUR FAMILY to give veggie noodles a try, this is the dish to serve them. However, you might want to double the recipe, as they will probably ask for second helpings.

MAKES 4 SERVINGS

In a large mixing bowl, combine the ground beef, Parmesan, almond flour, garlic powder, oregano, and the egg. Season with the salt and pepper. Using your hands, mix the ingredients until thoroughly combined. Shape into meatballs.

In a large skillet, heat the oil over medium-high heat. Add the meatballs and cook for 5 minutes, turning frequently, until evenly browned. Add the marinara and reduce the heat to low. Cover and cook for 15 minutes or until the meatballs are cooked through.

Add the squash, cover, and cook for 3 to 5 minutes until the squash is tender. Toss to coat. Top with the basil just before serving.

CALORIES 600 | PROTEIN 43 G (28%) | CARBS 18 G (12%) | FAT 40 G (60%)
SAT FAT 13 G | FIBER 6 G

1½ pounds lean ground beef

½ cup grated Parmesan cheese

½ cup almond flour

1 teaspoon garlic powder

1 teaspoon oregano

1 egg

Salt and freshly ground black pepper

1 tablespoon olive oil

2 cups no-sugar-added marinara

2 large yellow squash (about 1½ pounds), trimmed and spiralized into noodles

¼ cup fresh basil, chopped

DOUBLE CHEESE-STUFFED MEATBALLS

WHAT COULD POSSIBLY BE BETTER than a meatball? A meatball that's stuffed with two kinds of cheese! If you have time to do so, cover the meatballs and refrigerate for at least 30 minutes before cooking and they will be more likely to retain a round shape.

MAKES 4 SERVINGS

4 (1-ounce) mozzarella cheese "sticks"

¼ cup grated Parmesan cheese

1½ pounds lean ground beef

1 teaspoon garlic powder

1 teaspoon dried oregano

Salt and freshly ground black pepper

2 teaspoons olive oil

Slice each cheese "stick" into 4 equal pieces (you'll have 16 pieces). Place the Parmesan in a small bowl. Set aside.

In a bowl, combine the beef, Parmesan, garlic powder, and oregano. Season with the salt and pepper. Using your hands, mix the seasonings into the beef until thoroughly combined. Divide the beef into 16 equal lumps.

To make a meatball, press a piece of cheese into a portion of the beef and roll gently, taking care to ensure the cheese is thoroughly encased.

In a large skillet, warm the oil over medium-high heat. Working in batches, cook the meatballs, turning frequently, for 5 to 8 minutes or until cooked through and firm. Let rest a few minutes before serving.

CALORIES 460 | PROTEIN 45 G (40%) | CARBS 3 G (2%) | FAT 29 G (58%)
SAT FAT 12.3 G | FIBER 0 G

BETTER THAN MOM'S MEATLOAF

YOUR MOM'S MEATLOAF RECIPE probably included oatmeal or breadcrumbs, but you avoid those extra carbs in this version by using crumbled pork rinds in their place. An added bonus: The pork adds a subtle barbecue flavor to the finished dish. Serve with mashed cauliflower and a side of green beans.

MAKES 6 SERVINGS

Preheat the oven to 350°F. Brush a shallow baking dish with olive oil.

In a large mixing bowl, combine the beef, pork rinds, celery, onion, egg, tomato paste, parsley, and Parmesan. Season with the salt and pepper. Using your hands, mix the ingredients until thoroughly combined. Transfer the mixture to the prepared baking dish and shape it into a loaf.

Bake for 1 hour or until a thermometer inserted into the center of the loaf registers 145°F. Remove from the oven and let rest for 10 minutes to allow the juices to settle back into the loaf.

CALORIES 340 | PROTEIN 29 G (35%) | CARBS 5 G (6%) | FAT 22 G (59%)
SAT FAT 8.7 G | FIBER 1 G

1½ pounds lean ground beef

1 cup pork rinds, crumbled

1 rib celery, finely chopped

½ onion, finely chopped

1 egg

⅓ cup tomato paste

¼ cup chopped fresh parsley

½ cup grated Parmesan cheese

Salt and freshly ground black pepper

SLOW COOKER CHILI

HERE'S A DISH THAT IS PURE COMFORT on a cold day. Toss in a few red pepper flakes if you need a little extra heat.

1 pound lean ground beef

1 pound hot Italian sausage, casings removed

½ onion, chopped

½ red bell pepper, seeded and chopped

4 cloves garlic, minced

1 can (10-ounce) diced tomatoes with green chiles

1 can (6-ounce) tomato paste

1 tablespoon chili powder

1½ teaspoons ground cumin

½ cup Cheddar cheese

½ cup sour cream

4 scallions, thinly sliced

In a large skillet, brown the beef and sausage over medium-high heat, breaking up the meat as it cooks with the side of a spoon. Transfer the meat to a slow cooker. Add the onion, bell pepper, garlic, tomatoes, tomato paste, chili powder, and cumin. Mix until thoroughly combined. Cover and cook on HIGH for 6 hours or LOW for 8 hours. Serve topped with the Cheddar, sour cream, and the scallion slices.

CALORIES 575 | PROTEIN 40 G (28%) | CARBS 14 G (9%) | FAT 40 G (63%)
SAT FAT 15.8 G | FIBER 2 G

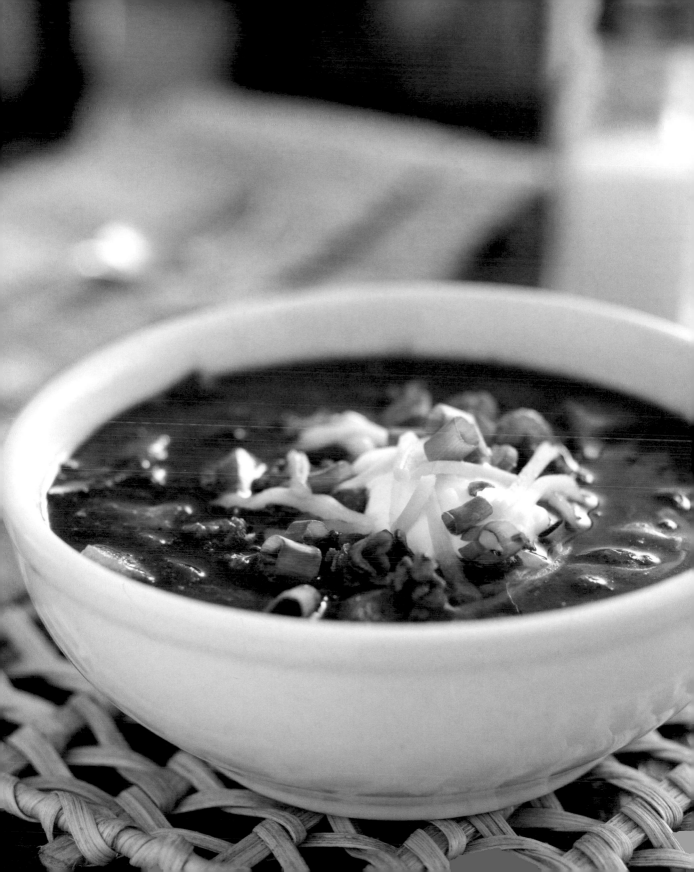

BEEF AND PEANUT STEW

MANY STEWS OWE THEIR THICKNESS to flour, potatoes, and other starchy vegetables that break down during the cooking process. This stew develops a luscious texture on its own with the addition of peanut butter and just the right amount of sweet potato.

MAKES 6 SERVINGS

2 pounds beef chuck, cut into cubes

Salt and freshly ground black pepper

1 teaspoon olive oil

1 quart reduced-sodium chicken broth

1 large sweet potato, peeled and chopped

1 onion, chopped

2 cloves garlic, minced

1 tablespoon red curry paste

3 tablespoons smooth peanut butter

4 cups chopped kale

1 cup cherry tomatoes, halved

½ cup chopped peanuts (optional)

½ cup chopped fresh cilantro (optional)

Season the beef with the salt and pepper. In a large skillet, warm the oil over medium-high heat. Cook the beef for 10 minutes until browned. Transfer the beef to the slow cooker. Add the broth, sweet potato, onion, garlic, and curry paste. Cover and cook on HIGH for 5 hours. Stir in the peanut butter, kale, and tomato halves. Cook 1 hour longer until the beef is fork tender. Sprinkle with the peanuts and cilantro just before serving (if using).

CALORIES 430 | PROTEIN 36 G (34%) | CARBS 12 G (11%) | FAT 26 G (55%)
SAT FAT 8.8 G | FIBER 2 G

BEEF KEBABS *with Chimichurri Sauce*

WARNING: This chimichurri sauce is positively addictive! It makes a wonderful accompaniment to just about any grilled meat you care to pair it with.

MAKES 4 SERVINGS

TO MAKE THE CHIMICHURRI: Combine the red onion, olive oil, vinegar, garlic, and oregano. Season to taste with the salt and pepper and add the red pepper flakes (if using). Refrigerate until you start grilling the kebabs (this part of the sauce can be made a few hours ahead). Just before serving whisk in the parsley and cilantro. Add the water, 1 tablespoon at a time, until the sauce reaches your desired thickness.

TO MAKE THE KEBABS: If using bamboo skewers, soak them in water at least 30 minutes before grilling. Prepare the grill (medium-high heat).

Season the meat with the salt and pepper. Thread the skewers with alternating pieces of beef, onion, zucchini, and tomatoes. Place the kebabs over direct heat and grill until the vegetables are tender and the beef reaches desired doneness, about 2 to 3 minutes per side for medium-rare. Transfer the kebabs to a platter and top with the chimichurri sauce.

CALORIES 465 | PROTEIN 33 G (28%) | CARBS 11 G (9%) | FAT 32 G (63%)
SAT FAT 9.1 G | FIBER 3 G

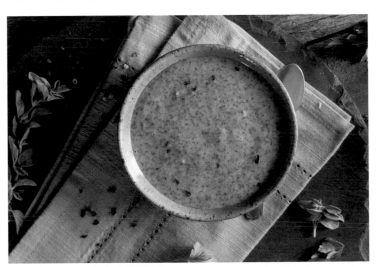

Chimichurri Sauce

¼ cup red onion, finely chopped

¼ cup extra-virgin olive oil

2 tablespoons cider vinegar

2 cloves garlic, chopped

1 teaspoon dried oregano

Salt and freshly ground black pepper

⅛ teaspoon red pepper flakes (optional)

¼ cup fresh parsley, finely chopped

¼ cup fresh cilantro, finely chopped

2 to 3 tablespoons water

Kebabs

1½ pounds sirloin, cut into 1 inch cubes

Salt and freshly ground black pepper

1 large red onion, cut into large chunks

2 small zucchini, sliced into large chunks

18 cherry tomatoes

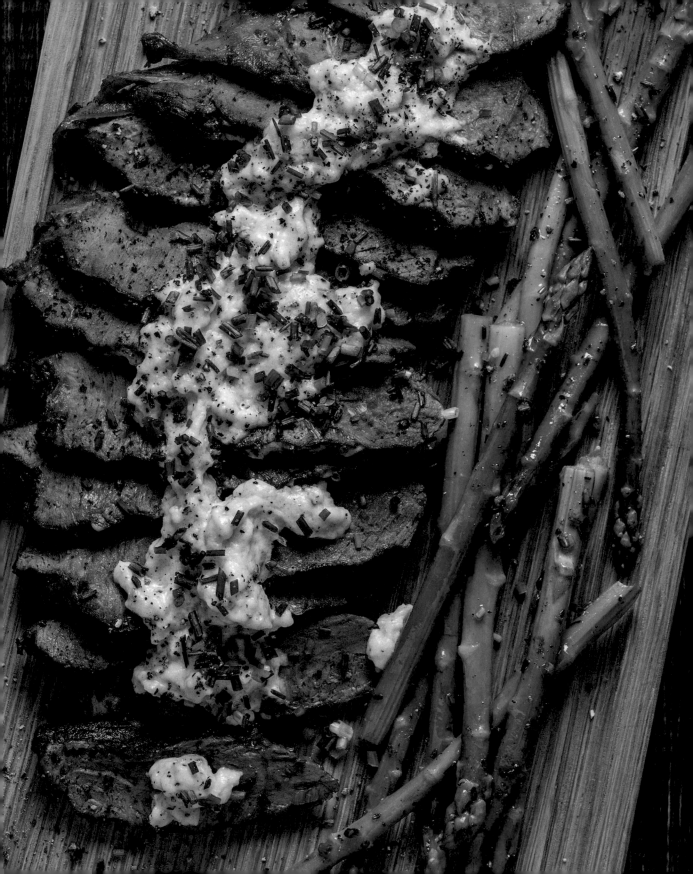

GRILLED SIRLOIN STEAKS
with Blue Cheese-Walnut Butter

THESE JUICY STEAKS are worthy of any special occasion, but they're so easy to prepare you may be tempted to make them more frequently. If you like, save a few minutes the next time you have a craving by making a double batch of the Blue Cheese—Walnut Butter portion of the recipe and storing leftovers in the freezer for up to 3 months.

MAKES 4 SERVINGS

Pat the steaks dry and place them in a large baking dish. Rub with 1 tablespoon of rosemary, the garlic, and a generous sprinkling of salt and pepper. Cover and let stand 1 hour at room temperature.

TO MAKE THE BUTTER: Toast the walnuts in a dry skillet over medium heat until fragrant, about 5 minutes. Tip onto a plate to let cool. Finely chop the walnuts and combine with the blue cheese, butter, the remaining rosemary, and parsley. Mash with a fork until thoroughly combined. Season to taste with salt and pepper and set aside.

Prepare the grill (medium-high heat). Cook the steaks to desired doneness, about 5 minutes per side for medium-rare. Transfer the steaks to a platter and let stand 5 minutes. Top each steak with a spoonful of the butter mixture, and sprinkle with the chives just before serving.

CALORIES 659 | PROTEIN 50 G (30.3%) | CARBS 2.6 G (1.6%) | FAT 49 G (66.9%)
SAT FAT 24 G | FIBER 1 G

4 (8 ounce) sirloin steaks

2 tablespoon chopped fresh rosemary, divided

1 tablespoon chopped garlic

Salt and freshly ground pepper

¼ cup walnuts

1 cup crumbled blue cheese

¼ cup (½ stick) unsalted butter at room temperature

1 tablespoon chopped fresh chives

CHORIZO-STUFFED ZUCCHINI

ONCE YOU GET THE HANG of how to assemble this dish, it's very easy to adapt to different flavor profiles. For example, you can create a simple Italian meal from the same basic recipe with a combination of Italian sausage and mozzarella, served on a bed of arugula.

MAKES 4 SERVINGS

2 large zucchini (about 1½ pounds), cut in half lengthwise

1 tablespoon olive oil

½ pound Mexican chorizo, chopped

½ large onion, finely chopped

1 or 2 serrano chiles, finely chopped (optional)

1 clove garlic, minced

2 Roma tomatoes

Salt and freshly ground black pepper

1 cup shredded Cheddar cheese

½ cup crushed pork rinds

Preheat the oven to 350°F. Brush a 9- x 13-inch baking dish with olive oil.

With a small spoon, scoop out the flesh of the zucchini leaving a ⅛- to ¼-inch thick shell. Set the zucchini shells aside and roughly chop the scooped-out flesh.

In a large skillet, warm the oil over medium heat. Cook the chorizo for 5 minutes, stirring occasionally, until browned (if using fresh, uncooked chorizo remove the casings and use the side of a spoon to break up the meat as it cooks). Stir in the chopped onion, serrano chiles (if using), and garlic and cook for 2 minutes longer, stirring occasionally. Reduce the heat to low and stir in the chopped zucchini flesh and the tomatoes. Season to taste with the salt and pepper. Cover and let simmer, stirring occasionally, for 8 to 10 minutes or until the chopped zucchini is tender. Remove from the heat.

Arrange the hollowed zucchini halves on the baking sheet, and fill each zucchini boat with equal amounts of the chorizo stuffing. Sprinkle the tops with the Cheddar and pork rinds.

Bake the stuffed zucchini for 20 to 25 minutes or until the zucchini is cooked through and the cheese has melted and browned.

CALORIES 465 | PROTEIN 25 G (21%) | CARBS 10 G (9%) | FAT 36 G (70%)
SAT FAT 14.6 G | FIBER 2 G

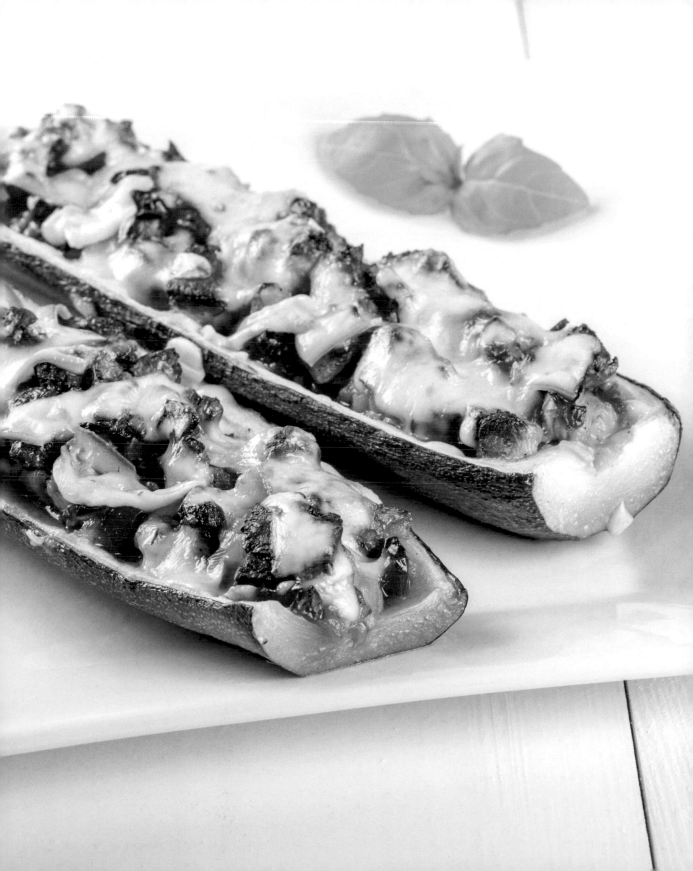

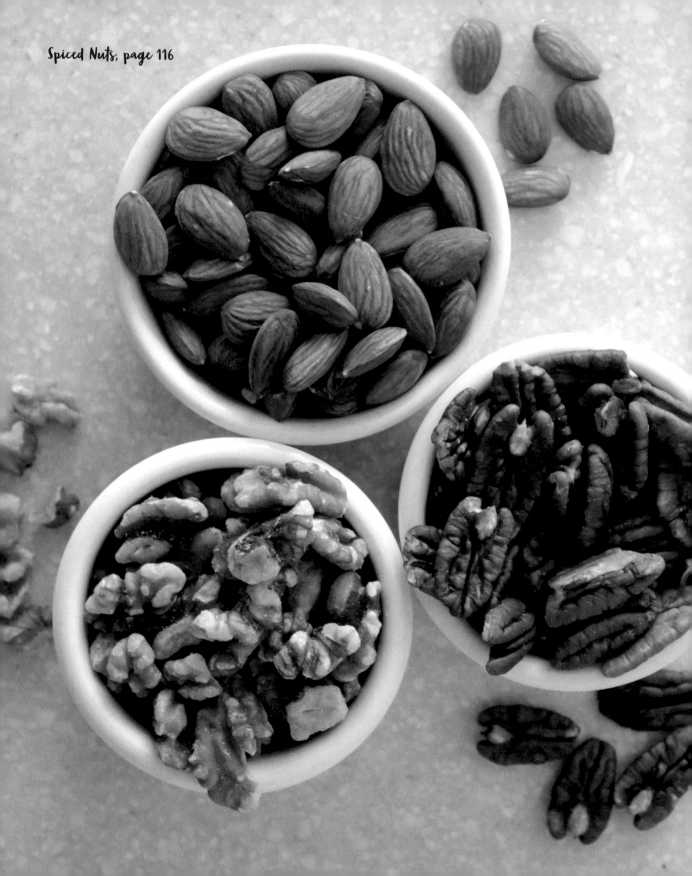

Spiced Nuts, page 116

chapter 5
SNACKS

SPICED NUTS

WHEN YOU'RE CRAVING a salty, spicy snack, these toasted nuts are the ticket. They're also nice additions to a salad instead of croutons.

MAKES 6 SERVINGS

1 teaspoon chili powder

½ teaspoon ground cumin

½ cup almonds

½ cup pecans

½ cup walnuts

1 tablespoon olive oil

Salt and freshly ground black pepper

In a small bowl, combine the chili powder and cumin. Set aside.

In a dry cast-iron skillet, toast the almonds, pecans, and walnuts over medium heat for 5 to 7 minutes, stirring occasionally, until fragrant and beginning to brown. Drizzle with the olive oil and add the spice mixture. Toss to coat. Season to taste with the salt and pepper. Let cool slightly before serving.

CALORIES 205 | PROTEIN 4 G (7%) | CARBS 5 G (9%) | FAT 20 G (84%)
SAT FAT 2 G | FIBER 3 G

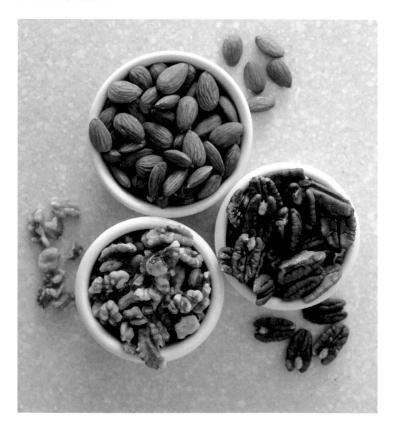

PARMESAN CRISPS

CRUNCHY. SALTY. SPICY. These keto-friendly crisps are remarkably similar to regular potato chips, but without the extra carbs.

MAKES 4 SERVINGS

Preheat the oven to 425°F. Line a baking sheet with parchment paper. Brush with olive oil.

Form 16 small mounds of Parmesan on the baking sheet (1 tablespoon each), placed at least 1 inch apart. Arrange the jalapeño slices on top of the Parmesan mounds. Top each mound with a piece of Provolone. Bake for 10 minutes until browned. Let cool, and store in a tightly sealed container for up to 3 days.

CALORIES 205 | PROTEIN 14 G (27%) | CARBS 4 G (8%) | FAT 15 G (65%)
SAT FAT 8.7 G | FIBER 0 G

1 cup grated Parmesan cheese

1 or 2 jalapeño peppers, sliced into 16 pieces

4 slices of Provolone cheese (about 4 ounces), quartered

PIMENTO-STUFFED CELERY

THIS RECIPE MAKES about 4 cups of pimento cheese, enough to feed a crowd or provide a few people with a steady supply of snacks for about a week.

MAKES 16 SERVINGS

½ cup mayonnaise

8 ounces cream cheese, softened

1 jar (4-ounce) diced pimiento, drained

1 teaspoon Worcestershire sauce

¼ teaspoon ground cayenne

2 cups shredded extra-sharp Cheddar cheese

2 cups shredded Gouda cheese

16 large ribs celery

In a large bowl, combine the mayonnaise, cream cheese, pimiento, Worcestershire sauce, and cayenne. Mix until thoroughly combined. Stir in the Cheddar and Gouda. Spoon about 2 tablespoons of the cheese mixture into a rib of celery just before serving until all ingredients are used. Leftovers can be stored in the refrigerator for up to 1 week.

CALORIES 220 | PROTEIN 8 G (15%) | CARBS 4 G (7%) | FAT 19 G (78%)
SAT FAT 8.8 G | FIBER 1 G

CAPRESE SKEWERS

ALL THE FLAVORS OF A FAVORITE SUMMER SALAD are even more fun when they're served on skewers. If you're putting these together as a party snack, try to make sure that your tomatoes and cheese balls are roughly the same size.

MAKES 6 SERVINGS

Place the mozzarella in a bowl and toss with the pesto. Thread the mozzarella, tomatoes, olives, and basil onto large toothpicks or bamboos skewers, alternating ingredients so that they are evenly distributed.

CALORIES 160 | PROTEIN 10 G (25%) | CARBS 5 G (13%) | FAT 11 G (62%)
SAT FAT 5 G | FIBER 1 G

8 ounces fresh mozzarella cheese balls, drained

2 tablespoons prepared pesto

2 cups grape or cherry tomatoes

½ cup pitted black olives

¼ cup fresh basil leaves

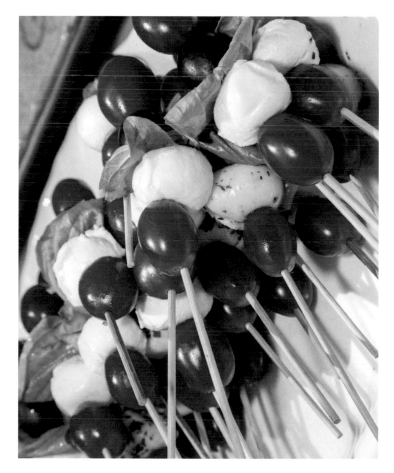

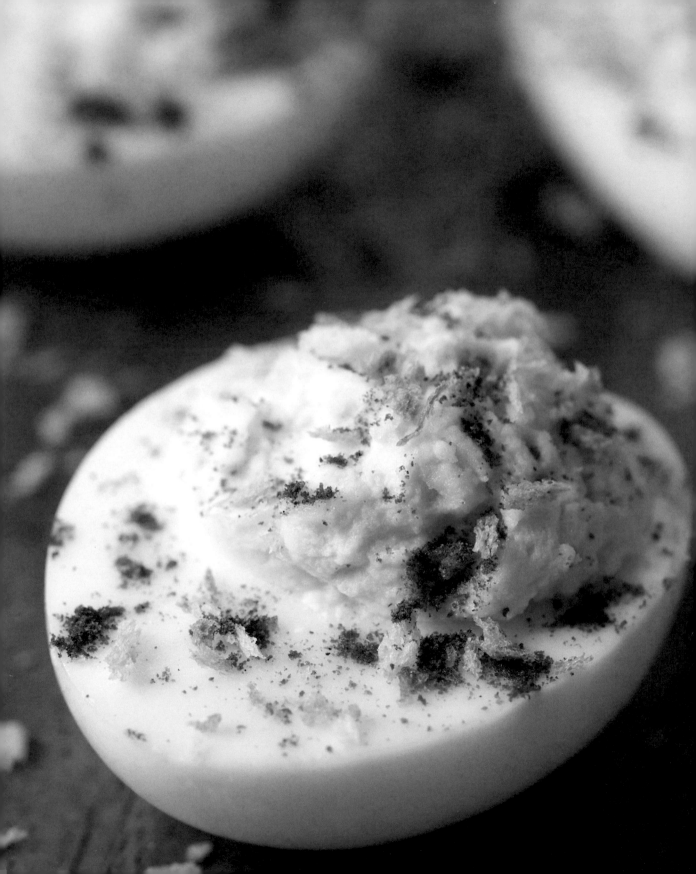

DEVILED EGGS

PERFECT FOR A PICNIC, mid-afternoon snack, or any time of day when a quick bite of protein hits the spot. If you prefer your deviled eggs with a bit more texture, consider substituting pickle relish for the mustard and a splash of pickle juice in place of the vinegar.

MAKES 4 SERVINGS

Slice the eggs in half lengthwise. Remove the yolks to a medium bowl and place the whites on a serving platter. Mash the yolks with a fork and add the mayonnaise, vinegar, and mustard, and mix well. Season to taste with the salt and pepper.

Spoon the yolk mixture into the egg whites. Sprinkle with the paprika and serve.

CALORIES 215 | PROTEIN 10 G (18%) | CARBS 1 G (2%) | FAT 19 G (80%)
SAT FAT 4.1 G | FIBER 0 G

6 hard-boiled eggs, peeled

¼ cup mayonnaise

1 teaspoon vinegar

1 teaspoon yellow mustard

Salt and freshly ground black pepper

Smoked paprika, for garnish

TUNA SALAD *on Cucumber*

INSTEAD OF CRACKERS, this recipe relies on the cool, refreshing crunch of a cucumber slice to support a delicious bite of tuna salad. Double the recipe for an easy, portable lunch option.

1 can (5-ounce) water-packed albacore tuna, drained

¼ cup mayonnaise

1 rib celery, finely chopped

1 tablespoon pickle relish

Salt and freshly ground black pepper

1 cucumber, peeled and sliced

2 tablespoons chia seeds

In a medium bowl, combine the tuna, mayonnaise, celery, and relish and stir until thoroughly combined. Season to taste with the salt and pepper. Arrange the cucumber slices on a serving plate and top with equal amounts of the tuna mixture. Sprinkle the chia seeds on top just before serving.

CALORIES 190 | PROTEIN 10 G (21%) | CARBS 6 G (13%) | FAT 14 G (66%)
SAT FAT 2.2 G | FIBER 3 G

CHUNKY GUACAMOLE
in Endive Cups

USING A PERFECTLY RIPE AVOCADO IS KEY to having the best guacamole. To test its readiness, squeeze gently. If it is ready to eat, it should yield slightly to pressure. While this snack is relatively high in carbs, it also packs a whopping 7 grams of fiber per serving.

MAKES 2 SERVINGS

Arrange the endive leaves on a serving plate. Finely chop any leftover interior leaves. Set aside.

In a medium bowl, mash the avocado with a fork or potato masher until chunky. Stir in the lime juice and season to taste with the salt and pepper. Add the tomato, scallion, cilantro, and chopped endive and stir until thoroughly combined. Spoon equal amounts of the guacamole into the endive cups just before serving.

CALORIES 130 | PROTEIN 2 G (5%) | CARBS 10 G (27%) | FAT 11 G (68%)
SAT FAT 1.5 G | FIBER 7 G

12 large endive leaves (from about 2 heads)

1 avocado, peeled

2 teaspoons fresh lime juice

Salt and freshly ground black pepper

1 small Roma tomato, finely chopped

1 scallion, finely chopped

2 tablespoons finely chopped fresh cilantro

BACON-WRAPPED JALAPEÑO POPPERS

GOING TO A PARTY and want to make sure there will be some keto-friendly foods you can eat? Bring these poppers to your next potluck and you'll be glad you did. But they're guaranteed to go fast, so set aside a few for yourself before you put the plate out.

MAKES 8 SERVINGS

½ pound lean ground beef

1 tablespoon Worcestershire sauce

Salt and freshly ground black pepper

16 jalapeño peppers, halved lengthwise and seeded

16 slices bacon, halved

4 ounces cream cheese

Preheat the oven to 400°F. Line a baking sheet with aluminum foil.

In a small skillet, brown the beef over medium-high heat for about 5 minutes, breaking up the meat with the side of a spoon as it cooks. Stir in the Worcestershire sauce during the last minute of cooking. Season to taste with the salt and pepper. Remove the skillet from the heat and allow to cool.

Spread a small amount of cream cheese inside each jalapeño half. Top with equal amounts of the ground beef. Carefully wrap a piece of bacon around each jalapeño half to enclose the filling.

Bake for 30 minutes until the bacon is crisp and the peppers have softened. Let cool before serving.

CALORIES 200 | PROTEIN 13 G (26%) | CARBS 3 G (6%) | FAT 15 G (68%)
SAT FAT 6.2 G | FIBER 1 G

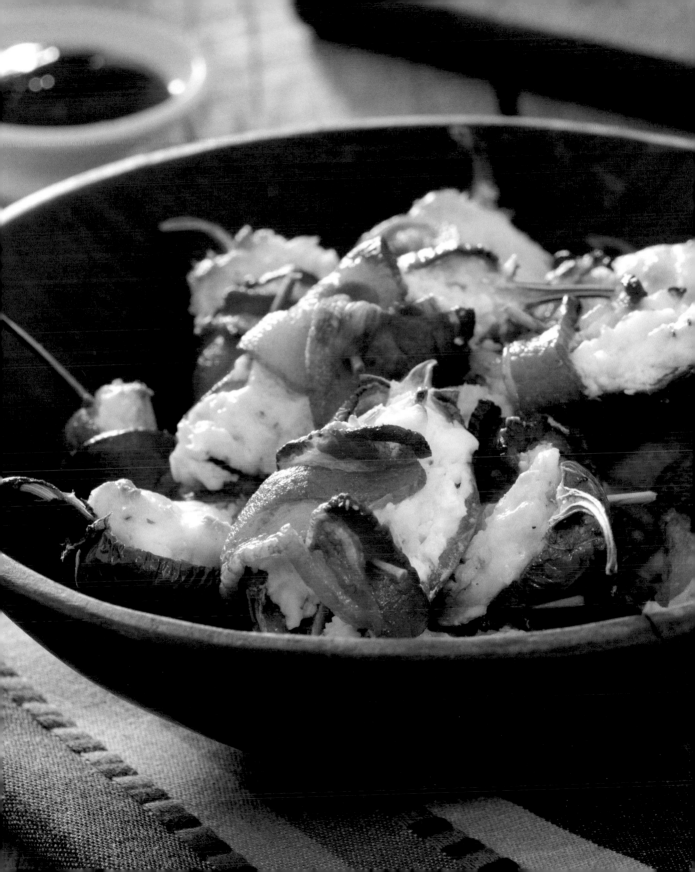

GOAT CHEESE AND ARTICHOKE DIP

THIS SAVORY DIP IS DELIGHTFUL as the centerpiece to a platter of raw veggies. Celery sticks, cucumber slices, bell pepper strips, and even endive spears are all perfect vessels for scooping. Should you be lucky enough to have any leftovers to refrigerate, consider folding a spoonful of this dip into tomorrow morning's breakfast omelet.

MAKES 8 SERVINGS

2 tablespoons olive oil

1 shallot, finely chopped

1 clove garlic, minced

1 can (14-ounce) artichoke hearts, packed in water, drained

8 ounces soft goat cheese, crumbled into large chunks

½ cup grated Parmesan cheese

1 tablespoon chopped fresh parsley

2 teaspoons fresh lemon juice

Salt and freshly ground black pepper

Dash of ground cayenne

In a small skillet, warm the oil over medium heat. Cook the shallot and garlic for 3 minutes until softened. Set aside.

In the work bowl of a food processor, combine the artichoke hearts, goat cheese, Parmesan, parsley, and lemon juice. Add the shallot mixture (remove all the oil from the bottom of the skillet). Process until smooth. Season to taste with the salt and pepper. Transfer the mixture to a serving bowl and sprinkle with the cayenne.

CALORIES 180 | PROTEIN 10 G (22%) | CARBS 6 G (13%) | FAT 13 G (65%)
SAT FAT 7.1 G | FIBER 3 G

HERBED CREAM CHEESE AND WALNUT DIP

THIS SUPER-SIMPLE DIP is a snap to put together. While you can serve it alongside any combination of fresh keto-friendly veggies, radishes are an especially attractive option.

MAKES 6 SERVINGS

Preheat the oven to 275°F. Spread the walnuts on a baking sheet and bake until fragrant and toasted, about 10 minutes. Reserve 1 tablespoon of the nuts for garnish.

In a bowl, combine the walnuts, cream cheese, and chives. Mix until thoroughly combined. Season to taste with the salt and pepper. Transfer the mixture to a serving bowl and drizzle on the walnut oil. Top with the reserved walnuts and serve with the radishes.

½ cup chopped walnuts, divided

8 ounces cream cheese, softened

1 tablespoon chopped fresh chives

Salt and freshly ground black pepper

1 tablespoon walnut oil

1½ cups sliced radishes

CALORIES 220 | PROTEIN 4 G (7%) | CARBS 4 G (7%) | FAT 22 G (86%)
SAT FAT 8.1 G | FIBER 1 G

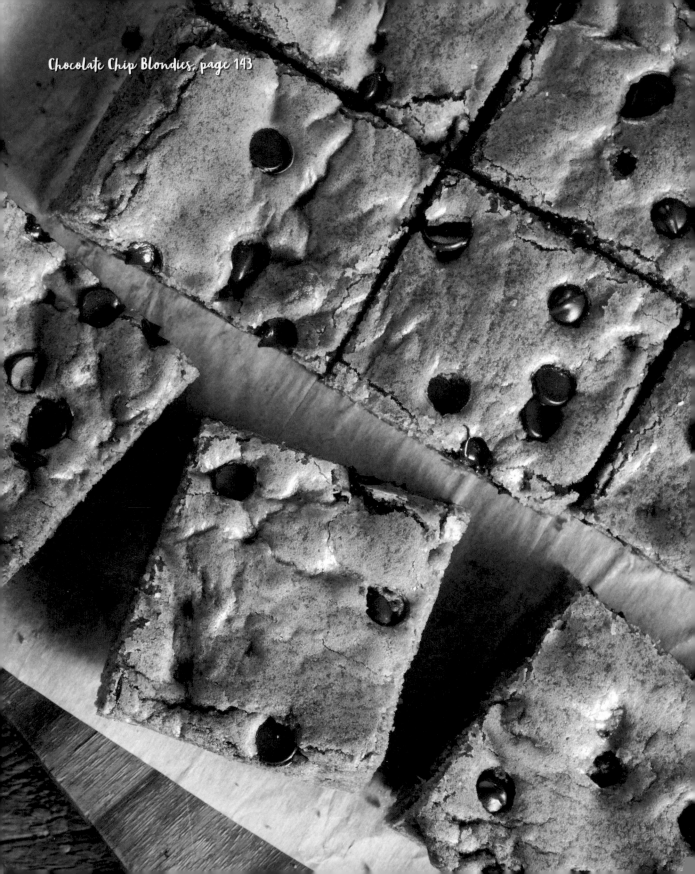

Chocolate Chip Blondies, page 143

chapter 6
DESSERTS

COCONUT PUDDING

RICH AND CREAMY AND OH SO SATISFYING, this pudding requires a few minutes on the stovetop, but once you taste the results you'll consider it time well spent.

MAKES 12 SERVINGS

1½ cups Swerve or another zero-carb granulated sweetener

1 cup unsweetened shredded coconut

1 cup heavy cream, divided

2 eggs

1 cup coconut milk

8-ounces cream cheese, cut into pieces

2 teaspoons coconut extract

½ teaspoon vanilla extract

In a large microwavable bowl, combine the sweetener, coconut, and ½ cup of the heavy cream. Microwave on HIGH for 1 minute. Set aside.

In another bowl, combine the remaining ½ cup of heavy cream and the eggs. Beat until thoroughly combined. Set aside.

In a medium pot, warm the coconut milk and cream cheese over medium heat. Whisk slowly, about 5 minutes, until the cream cheese has melted. Add the coconut and egg mixtures and continue whisking as the pudding cooks, about 5 minutes longer until bubbles form at the edge of the pot and the pudding begins to thicken. Remove from the heat and stir in the coconut and vanilla extract. Transfer the mixture to a large bowl. Let cool a bit, then cover and refrigerate at least 4 hours or preferably overnight.

CALORIE 215 | PROTEIN 3 G (6%) | CARBS 4 G (7%) | FAT 21 G (87%) | SAT FAT 14.1 G FIBER 0 G

RASPBERRY PUDDING

THE BEAUTY OF THIS DESSERT is that it calls for just five ingredients. But one taste and you'd never know it! While this dish is considered keto-friendly, it still has quite a few carbs (as well as fiber), so do measure your portion carefully.

MAKES 4 SERVINGS

Place the coconut milk, raspberries, and water in a blender and whirl until smooth. Transfer to a medium bowl. Stir in the chia seeds and vanilla extract. Cover and refrigerate overnight before serving.

CALORIES 213 | PROTEIN 4 G (7%) | CARBS 15 G (26%) | FAT 17 G (67%)
SAT FAT 11.2 G | FIBER 9 G

1 cup coconut milk

1 cup frozen raspberries

½ cup water

½ cup chia seeds

2 teaspoons vanilla extract

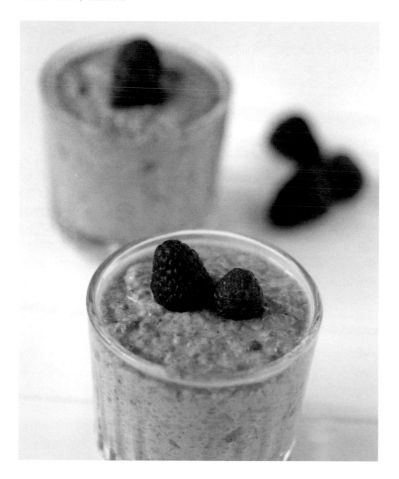

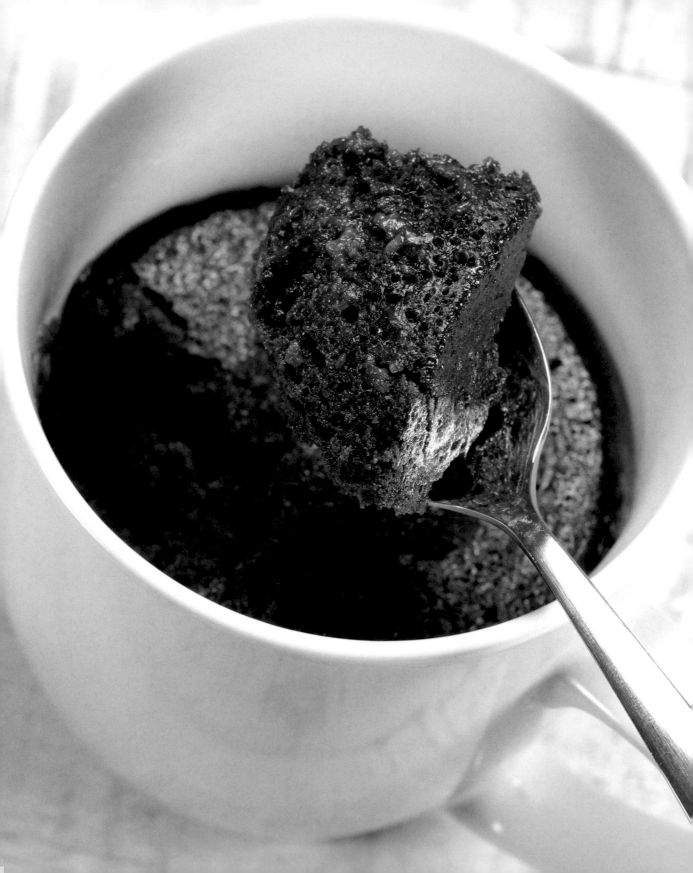

BEYOND DECADENT CHOCOLATE MUG CAKE

MICROWAVE OVEN HEATING levels vary, which can make a difference in a delicate, quick-cooking cake like this. Start with the lowest possible time and add 10 seconds in increments if you want your cake a little drier.

MAKES 2 SERVINGS

In a small bowl, combine the coconut flour, cocoa, sweetener, and baking powder. Stir until thoroughly combined.

Place the butter in the mug. Microwave on HIGH for 20 to 30 seconds until the butter is melted. Add the cream and the egg. Beat with a fork until thoroughly combined. Stir in the flour mixture and the vanilla extract.

Microwave on HIGH for 2½ to 3 minutes until the center is done and the top springs back when pressed. Let sit for several minutes. Run a knife around the inside edge of the mug to loosen the cake and gently transfer it to a plate. Slice in half. Serve warm topped with unsweetened whipped cream (if using).

CALORIES 220 | PROTEIN 5 G (9%) | CARBS 5 G (9%) | FAT 20 G (82%)
SAT FAT 11.6 G | FIBER 1 G

2 tablespoons coconut flour

2 tablespoons unsweetened cocoa

2 tablespoons Swerve or another granulated zero carb sweetener

½ teaspoon baking powder

2 tablespoons butter

2 tablespoons heavy cream

1 egg

1 teaspoon vanilla extract

½ cup whipped cream (optional)

NO-BAKE CHOCOLATE BALLS

THE TASTY MORSELS ARE PERFECT to have on hand for a quick midday snack. Plus, no-bake means no hassle!

MAKES 14 SERVINGS (2 BALLS PER SERVING)

⅓ cup Swerve or another zero-carb granulated sweetener

½ cup milk

½ cup butter

¼ teaspoon salt

¼ cup unsweetened cocoa powder

⅔ cup smooth peanut butter

½ cup sesame seeds

½ cup toasted pecans

1½ cup unsweetened shredded coconut, divided

1 teaspoon vanilla extract

In a medium pot, bring the sweetener, milk, butter, salt, and cocoa to a full boil over medium-high heat. Remove from the heat. Add the peanut butter and stir until melted. Stir in the sesame seeds, pecans, 1 cup of coconut, and the vanilla extract. Mix until thoroughly combined. By the tablespoon, make a ball and roll it in the remaining ½ cup of coconut. Refrigerate until firm.

CALORIES 250 | PROTEIN 5 G (8%) | CARBS 8 G (12%) | FAT 23 G (80%)
SAT FAT 10.2 G | FIBER 3 G

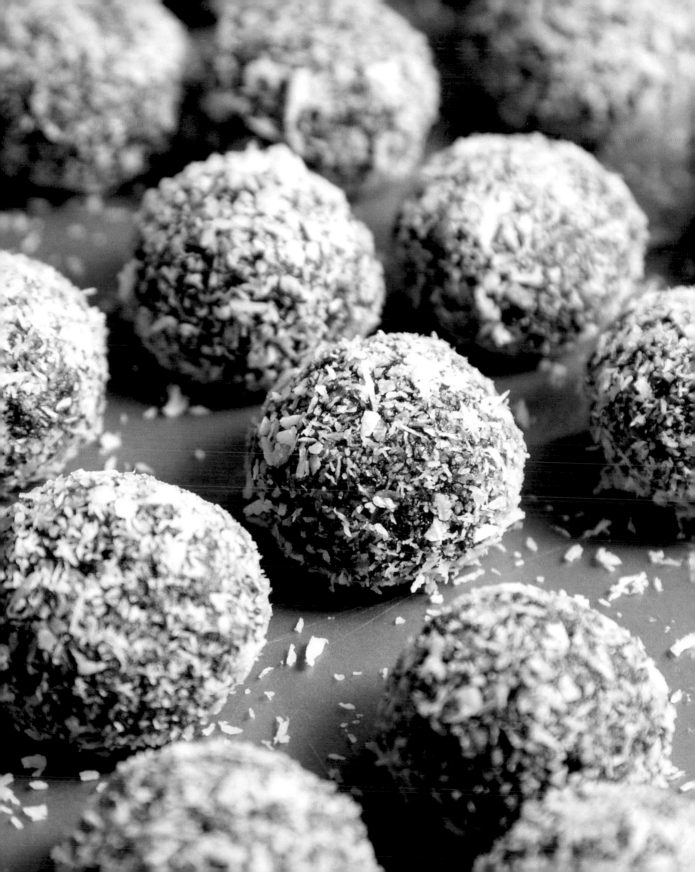

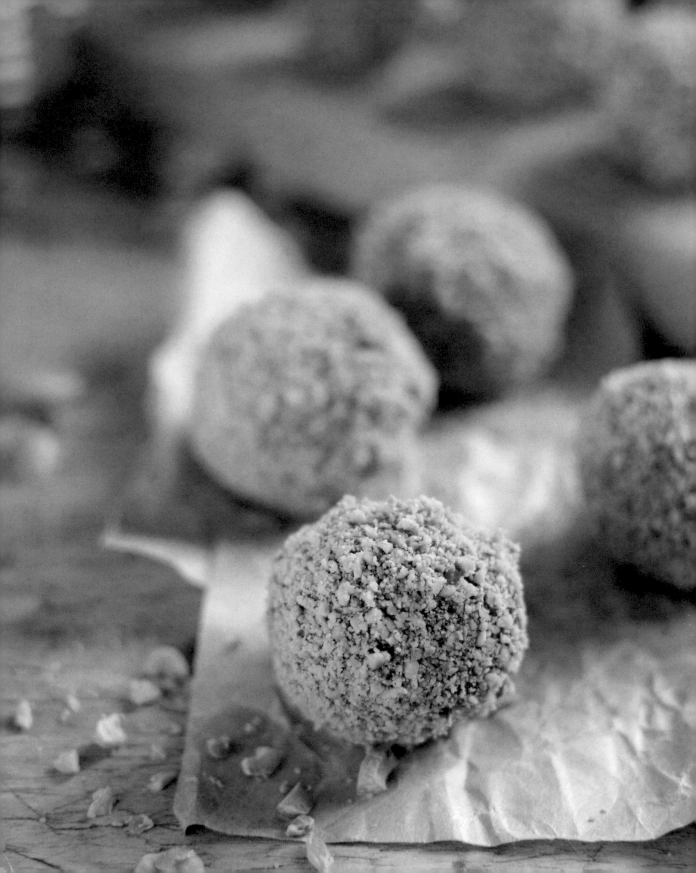

NO-BAKE PEANUT BUTTER BITES

THESE SUPER-NUTTY CONFECTIONS hit the spot when you want something sweet and salty. For a bit more decadence, consider melting some extra-dark, sugar-free chocolate to drizzle on top.

In a large bowl, combine the peanut butter, almond flour, sweetener, and vanilla extract. Mix well, using your hands, if necessary. Form the mixture into a ball and refrigerate until firm. Shape into 16 balls and roll in the chopped peanuts to coat.

CALORIES 155 | PROTEIN 6 G (14%) | CARBS 6 G (14%) | FAT 14 G (72%)
SAT FAT 2.2 G | FIBER 2 G

1 cup smooth peanut butter

1 cup almond flour

¼ cup Swerve or another zero-carb granulated sweetener

1 teaspoon vanilla extract

½ cup chopped peanuts

MOM'S BEST PEANUT BUTTER COOKIES

THESE CLASSIC COOKIES ARE SURPRISINGLY EASY to make keto-friendly. Tuck some into your next picnic or packed lunch and you're sure to put a smile on someone's face.

MAKES 8 SERVINGS (3 COOKIES EACH)

½ cup coconut flour

1 cup Swerve or another zero-carb granulated sweetener

1 cup smooth peanut butter

3 eggs

¼ teaspoon salt

1 teaspoon vanilla extract

Preheat the oven to 350°F. Line a baking sheet with parchment paper.

In a large bowl, combine the coconut flour, sweetener, peanut butter, eggs, salt, and vanilla extract. Mix until thoroughly combined.

By the tablespoon, roll the dough into portions and arrange on the baking sheet. Use the back of a fork to flatten the cookies slightly and make a distinct crisscross pattern. Bake for 15 to 17 minutes until the edges are golden brown. Transfer to a rack and let cool before serving.

CALORIES 225 | PROTEIN 10 G (16%) | CARBS 8 G (13%) | FAT 19 G (71%)
SAT FAT 4.1 G | FIBER 2 G

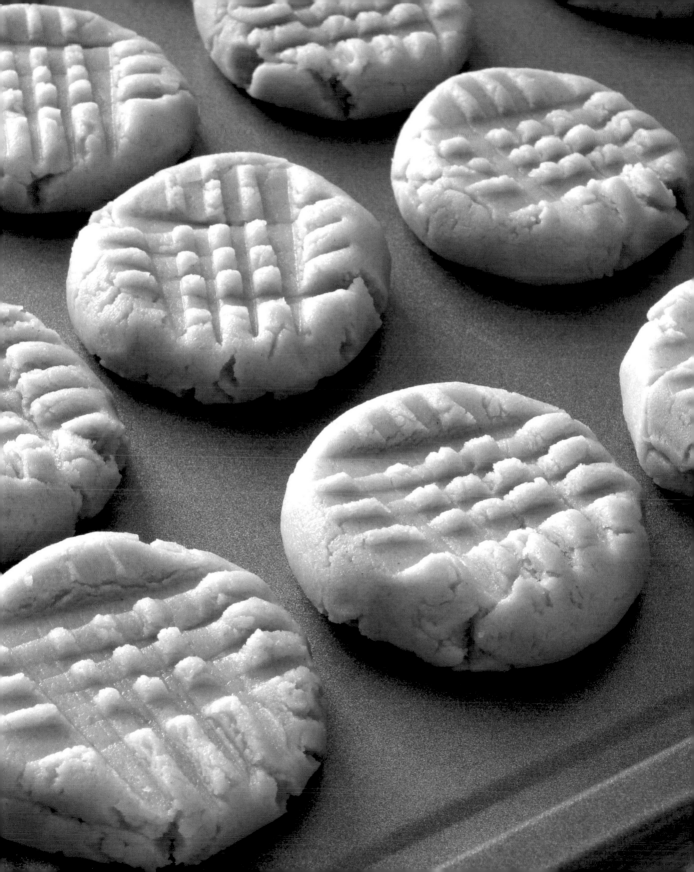

CAFÉ COOKIES

THESE SLIGHTLY SWEETENED COOKIES, with crunchy edges and a soft center, are the perfect companion to your midday cuppa joe. They expand quite a bit during baking, so plan accordingly.

MAKES 9 SERVINGS (2 COOKIES EACH)

1½ cups almond flour

1 tablespoon instant coffee powder

½ teaspoon baking soda

½ teaspoon salt

¼ teaspoon ground cinnamon

½ cup butter, softened

⅓ cup Swerve or another zero-carb granulated sweetener

2 eggs, separated

2 teaspoons vanilla extract

10 drops liquid stevia

Preheat the oven to 350°F. Line two baking sheets with parchment paper.

In a large bowl, combine the almond flour, coffee powder, baking soda, salt, and cinnamon. Stir until thoroughly combined. Set aside.

In another large bowl, use a mixer to cream the butter and sweetener until smooth. Add the egg yolks, vanilla extract, and stevia. Beat the butter mixture until fluffy. Add the flour mixture to the butter mixture and stir until well combined.

In another bowl, beat the egg whites on high speed until soft peaks form. Carefully fold the egg whites into the cookie batter. By the spoonful, place the dough onto the baking sheets and bake for 12 to 15 minutes until brown. Let cool on the baking sheets for a few minutes, then carefully transfer to a rack to finish cooling.

CALORIES 250 | PROTEIN 7 G (11%) | CARBS 6 G (9%) | FAT 23 G (80%) | SAT FAT 7.7 G
FIBER 3 G

PECAN-TOFFEE BARS

WITH A SHORTBREAD BASE and a rich, toffee topping enrobing the pecans, these are the holiday favorites that you remember. In fact, you may be delighted to slip these onto the dessert table and see the reaction of others when you tell them this is what low-carb baking tastes like.

MAKES 16 SERVINGS

Preheat the oven to 350°F. Line an 8- x 8-inch baking pan with parchment paper.

In the work bowl of a food processor, combine the almond flour, ¼ cup sweetener, ¼ cup butter, and the salt. Pulse until the mixture is a fine crumb. Press the mixture into the bottom and sides of the baking pan. Bake for 12 to 15 minutes until the edges begin to brown. Remove from the oven and let cool while assembling the topping.

In a heavy-bottomed pot, heat the remaining ½ cup butter and ¾ cup sweetener over medium heat, stirring until the sweetener is dissolved. Stop stirring and bring the mixture to a boil; cook for 5 to 7 minutes until the syrup becomes amber-colored. Stir in the vanilla extract.

Scatter the pecans evenly on top of the crust and pour the syrup over the pecans. Sprinkle with a pinch of the sea salt. Bake again for 15 to 20 minutes until the topping is dark and bubbling. Let cool completely before cutting into bars.

CALORIES 280 | PROTEIN 4 G (5%) | CARBS 5 G (7%) | FAT 29 G (88%) | SAT FAT 7.2 G
FIBER 3 G

1¼ cups almond flour

1 cup Swerve or another granulated zero-carb sweetener, divided

¾ cup butter, divided

¼ teaspoon salt

½ teaspoon vanilla extract

3 cups chopped pecans

Pinch of sea salt

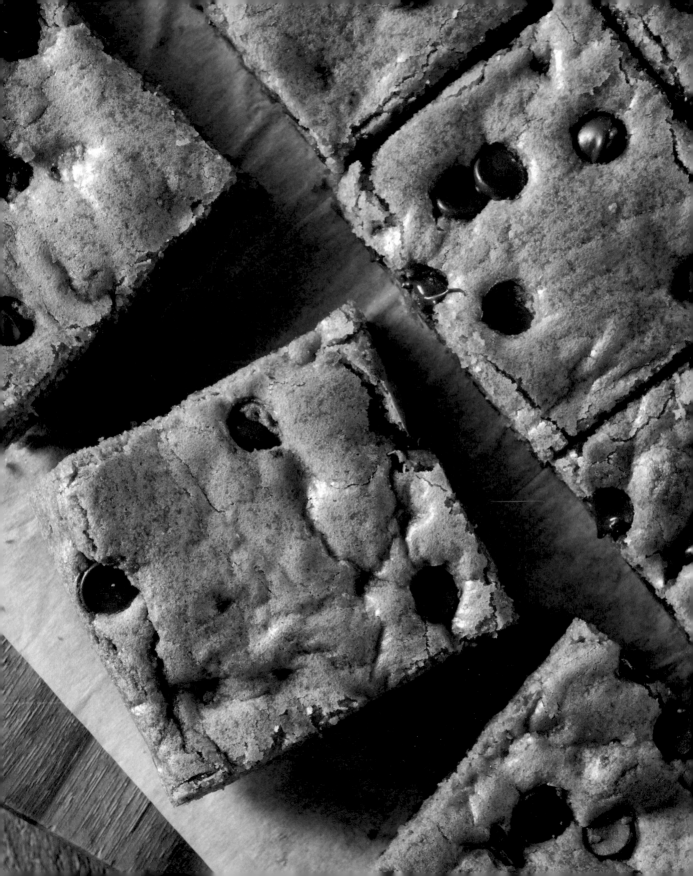

CHOCOLATE CHIP BLONDIES

BLONDIES ARE A WONDERFUL HYBRID, something like a cookie yet easy to bake, like a brownie. In fact, you could make about 1 dozen cookies from this recipe if you choose to portion them out onto a baking sheet. Either way, this is a recipe you're likely to turn to again and again.

MAKES 9 SERVINGS

Preheat the oven to 350°F. Line an 8- x 8-inch baking pan with parchment paper.

In a large bowl, combine the almond flour, baking powder, and salt. Stir until thoroughly combined. Set aside.

In another large bowl, use a mixer to cream the butter, sweetener, and molasses until smooth. Add the egg and vanilla extract. Beat the butter mixture until fluffy. Add the flour mixture to the butter mixture and stir until well combined. Stir in the chocolate chips.

Transfer the dough to the baking pan and bake for 20 to 25 minutes until golden brown. Remove from the oven and let cool completely before slicing

CALORIES 290 | PROTEIN 5 G (7%) | CARBS 6 G (9%) | FAT 25 G (84%) | SAT FAT 10.1 G
FIBER 4 G

2 cups almond flour

1 teaspoon baking powder

½ teaspoon salt

½ cup butter, softened

½ cup Swerve or another granulated zero-carb sweetener

2 teaspoons molasses

1 egg

1 teaspoon vanilla extract

½ cup sugar-free chocolate chips

STRAWBERRY FROZEN DESSERT

YOU MIGHT WANT TO DOUBLE THIS RECIPE if you're at peak strawberry season right now. If the dessert is especially hard after freezing, let it sit at room temperature before serving until it reaches the ideal consistency.

MAKES 4 SERVINGS

2 cups sliced strawberries

1¼ cups sour cream

¼ cup Swerve or another granulated zero-carb sweetener

¼ cup coconut oil

1 teaspoon vanilla extract

¼ teaspoon salt

In the work bowl of a food processor, combine the strawberries, sour cream, sweetener, coconut oil, vanilla extract, and salt. Whirl until smooth.

Transfer the mixture to an ice cream maker and process following the manufacturer's instructions. Freeze in a tightly sealed container until ready to serve.

CALORIES 285 | PROTEIN 2 G (3%) | CARBS 9 G (12%) | FAT 28 G (85%) | SAT FAT 20.1 FIBER 2 G

LIME-AVOCADO ICE CREAM

IF YOU HAVE AN ICE CREAM MAKER, you'll love making your own sugar-free, dairy-free desserts. This particular creation is pure refreshment on a hot day.

MAKES 6 SERVINGS

In the work bowl of a food processor, combine the avocado, sweetener, lime juice, almond extract, and salt. Mix until smooth. Continue running the food processor and slowly add the almond milk and whirl until thoroughly combined.

Transfer the mixture to an ice cream maker and process following the manufacturer's instructions. Freeze in a tightly sealed container until ready to serve.

CALORIES 125 | PROTEIN 2 G (6%) | CARBS 6 G (18%) | FAT 11 G (76%) | SAT FAT 1.4 G
FIBER 5 G

3 avocados, peeled

¾ cup Swerve or another granulated zero-carb sweetener

2 tablespoons fresh lime juice

1 teaspoon almond extract

½ teaspoon salt

2 cups unsweetened almond milk

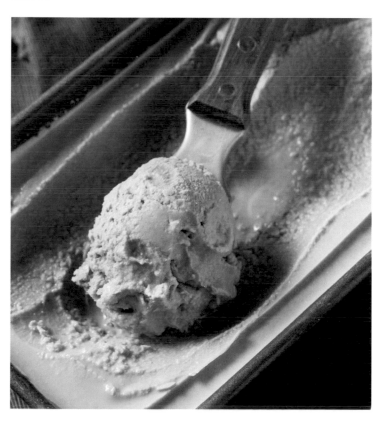

RICH CHOCOLATE MOUSSE

THIS IS THE ULTIMATE DECADENT DESSERT to serve after a dinner party. Plus the flavors improve with a little time in the fridge, so it's a make-ahead solution that lets you enjoy more time with guests.

MAKES 6 SERVINGS

8 ounces cream cheese, softened

⅓ cup + 1 teaspoon Swerve or another granulated zero-carb sweetener, divided

¼ cup unsweetened cocoa powder

3 tablespoons sour cream

2 tablespoons butter, softened

1 tablespoon instant coffee powder

2 teaspoons vanilla extract, divided

⅔ cup heavy cream

In the work bowl of a food processor, combine the cream cheese, ⅓ cup of the sweetener, the cocoa, sour cream, butter, coffee powder, and 1 teaspoon vanilla extract. Pulse until smooth. Transfer to a large bowl.

In another large bowl, whip the heavy cream until soft peaks form. Add the remaining teaspoon of vanilla extract and the teaspoon of sweetener. Whip again until stiff peaks form.

Carefully fold half of the whipped cream into the chocolate mixture until thoroughly combined. Repeat with the remaining whipped cream. Transfer to serving dishes, cover, and refrigerate until ready to serve.

CALORIES 285 | PROTEIN 4 G (6%) | CARBS 5 G (7%) | FAT 28 G (87%) | SAT FAT 16.4 G FIBER 1 G

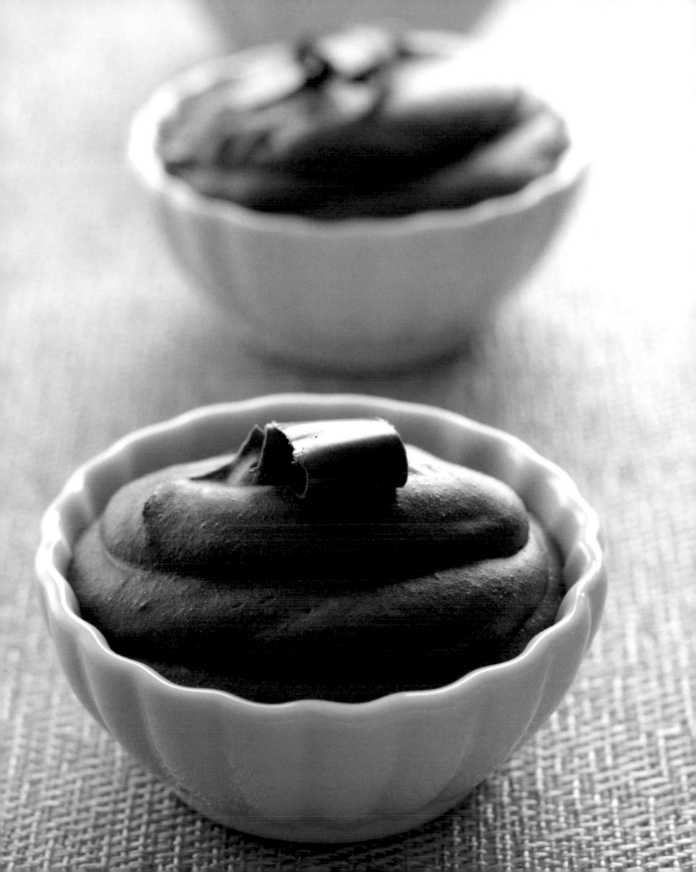

SOY GOOD CHOCOLATE PIE

YOU'D NEVER GUESS THAT TOFU is a main ingredient in the filling of this splurge-worthy creation, because all you taste is intense chocolate goodness. With only 4 grams of carbs per serving, it's a keto-friendly keeper.

MAKES 12 SERVINGS

½ cup walnuts

2 tablespoons Swerve or another granulated zero-carb sweetener

1 cup almond flour

⅓ cup golden flax meal

⅓ cup vanilla whey protein powder

⅛ teaspoon salt

6 tablespoons butter, melted

12 ounces silken extra-firm tofu, drained, patted dry

1½ cups sugar-free chocolate chips, melted

½ cup coconut milk

2 tablespoons coconut oil

1 teaspoon vanilla extract

Preheat the oven to 350°F.

In the work bowl of a food processor, combine the walnuts and sweetener. Pulse into fine crumbs. Transfer to a large bowl. Add the almond flour, flax meal, protein powder, salt, and butter. Stir with a fork until thoroughly combined. The mixture should hold its shape when squeezed firmly; if not, add a bit more butter. Transfer the mixture to a 9-inch pie plate and press firmly into the bottom and sides of the plate. Poke the bottom of the crust with the tines of a fork in several places. Bake for 10 minutes until set. Let cool completely and wipe out the work bowl before proceeding to the next step.

In the work bowl of the food processor, combine the tofu, chocolate, coconut milk, coconut oil, and vanilla extract. Process until smooth. Pour the mixture into the cooled pie crust. Cover and refrigerate at least 4 hours until set, preferably overnight.

CALORIES 350 | PROTEIN 7 G (10%) | CARBS 4 G (5%) | FAT 28 G (85%)
SAT FAT 14.2 G | FIBER 4 G

CREAMY LEMON CHEESECAKE BARS

THESE TART, CREAMY LITTLE CHEESECAKE BARS are the perfect way to finish a special Sunday supper. If you aren't a lemon fan, try another flavor of sugar-free gelatin, like cherry, orange, raspberry, or lime.

MAKES 9 SERVINGS

Preheat the oven to 350°F.

In the work bowl of a food processor, whirl the pecans and sweetener until the nuts are finely ground. Transfer the nuts to a large bowl and add the almond flour and butter. Stir with a fork until thoroughly combined. The mixture should hold its shape when squeezed firmly; if not, add a bit more butter. Transfer the mixture to a 9- x 9-inch baking dish and press firmly into the bottom. Poke with the tines of a fork in several places. Bake for 15 minutes until set. Let cool completely and wipe out the work bowl before proceeding to the next step.

Fill a microwavable measuring cup with 1 cup of water. Microwave on HIGH for 2 minutes until the water is boiling. Add the gelatin and stir until thoroughly combined. Let cool to room temperature.

In the work bowl of the food processor, combine the cream cheese, ricotta, lemon juice, and zest and process until the cheeses are thoroughly combined. With the food processor still running, add the gelatin to the cheese mixture in a slow, steady stream. Process until smooth, stopping to scrape the work bowl if necessary. Pour the mixture into the cooled nut crust, cover, and chill at least 4 hours until set.

CALORIES 310 | PROTEIN 8 G (10%) | CARBS 6 G (7%) | FAT 30 G (83%)
SAT FAT 11.4 G | FIBER 2 G

1 cup pecans

2 tablespoons Swerve or another granulated zero-carb sweetener

¾ cup almond flour

¼ cup butter, melted

1 cup boiling water

1 (0.3-ounce) package sugar-free lemon gelatin

8 ounces cream cheese, softened

1 cup ricotta cheese

2 tablespoons fresh lemon juice

1 tablespoon lemon zest

CREAMY CHEESECAKE
with Blueberry Sauce

LOW-CARB CHEESECAKE IS A REALITY—and you don't need to give up that satisfying crust! The secret: pecans plus almond flour. When it comes to the sweet fruit finishing touch, low-glycemic blueberries are perfect for a ketogenic weight loss plan. If you prefer, substitute with strawberries instead.

MAKES 12 SERVINGS

Cheesecake

1 cup pecans

1 cup almond flour

1 cup Swerve or another granulated zero-carb sugar replacement, divided

1 cup vanilla whey protein isolate powder

4 tablespoons unsalted butter, melted

2 (8 ounce) packages cream cheese, softened

1 tablespoon vanilla extract

½ cup heavy cream

Fresh mint (for garnish)

Blueberry Sauce

2 cups blueberries, frozen or fresh

2 tablespoons Swerve sugar replacement

2 tablespoons water

2 teaspoons fresh lemon juice

Pinch of nutmeg

TO MAKE THE CHEESECAKE: In a dry skillet, toast the pecans over medium heat until fragrant. Tip onto a plate to let cool.

Combine the pecans, almond flour, ⅔ cup of sweetener, and the protein powder in the work bowl of a food processor and pulse until finely ground. Transfer the mixture to a large bowl and add the butter. Mix with a fork until thoroughly combined. Transfer the nut mixture into a pie plate and use the heel of your hand or the flat bottom of a measuring cup to press mixture evenly into the bottom and sides of the plate.

Rinse out the large bowl and add the cream cheese, remaining ⅓ cup of sweetener, and the vanilla extract. Beat with a hand mixer on high speed until smooth, stopping to scrape the side of the bowl as needed. In a small bowl, beat the heavy cream with a hand mixer until it is very stiff. Use a silicone spatula to gently fold half of the whipped cream into the cream cheese mixture. Repeat with remaining whipped cream. Transfer cream cheese mixture to the pie plate and spread evenly over the nut mixture. Cover with plastic wrap and refrigerate overnight. Top with the blueberry sauce and garnish with mint before serving.

TO MAKE THE BLUEBERRY SAUCE: Combine the blueberries, sweetener, water, and lemon juice in a small pan over medium-high heat. When the mixture begins to boil, reduce heat to low and continue cooking, stirring occasionally, until berries begin to burst and the mixture starts to thicken, about 10 minutes. Remove from heat and stir in the nutmeg. Let cool before serving.

CALORIES 354 | PROTEIN 8 G (9.0%) | CARBS 10 G (11.3%) | FAT 33 G (83.9%)
SAT FAT 13 G | FIBER 3 G

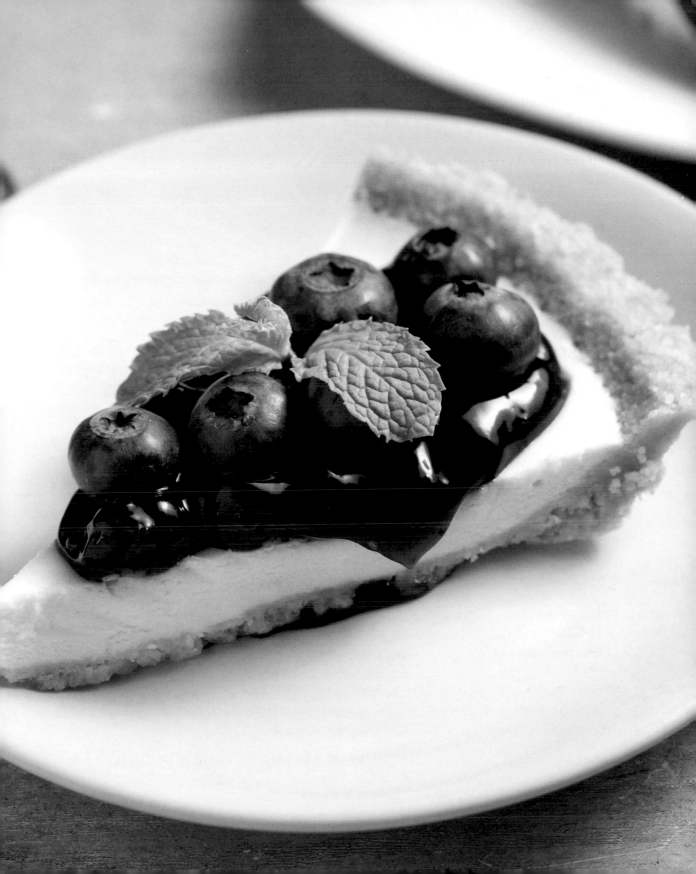

STRAWBERRY ICEBOX PIE

LIGHT, LUSCIOUS, AND OH SO EASY to put together. This is the recipe to celebrate the arrival of spring!

MAKES 10 SERVINGS

1 cup Swerve or another granulated zero-carb sweetener, divided

¾ cup unsweetened shredded coconut

¾ cup almond flour

6 tablespoons butter, melted

2½ cups sliced strawberries, divided

8 ounces cream cheese, softened

1 cup heavy cream

1 teaspoon vanilla extract

Preheat the oven to 350°F.

In a large bowl, combine ½ cup of the sweetener, the coconut, almond flour, and butter. Stir with a fork until thoroughly combined. The mixture should hold its shape when squeezed firmly; if not, add a bit more butter. Transfer the mixture to a pie plate and press firmly into the bottom and sides of the plate. Poke with the tines of a fork in several places. Bake for 15 minutes until set. Let cool completely while proceeding to the next step.

In the work bowl of a food processor, combine 2 cups of the strawberries, the remaining ½ cup of sweetener, and the cream cheese. Process until very smooth, stopping to scrape down the bowl as necessary. Transfer the strawberry mixture to a large bowl.

In another bowl, combine the cream and vanilla extract. Beat with a mixer until stiff peaks form. Carefully fold half of the whipped cream into the strawberry mixture until thoroughly combined. Repeat with the remaining whipped cream. Transfer to the pie plate, cover, and freeze until firm. About 30 minutes before serving, remove the pie from the freezer. Top with the remaining cup of strawberry slices.

CALORIES 315 | PROTEIN 4 G (5%) | CARBS 8 G (10%) | FAT 31 G (85%) | SAT FAT 18 G
FIBER 3 G

WALNUT-BERRY CRISP

BLUEBERRIES, BLACKBERRIES, RASPBERRIES, OR STRAWBERRIES—any combination of fruit serves well in this easy-to-prepare crisp. In fact, it is so good you might even be tempted to enjoy any leftovers for breakfast.

MAKES 8 SERVINGS

Preheat the oven to 350°F. Brush an 8- x 8-inch baking pan with olive oil.

Place the berries in the bottom of the baking dish. Sprinkle the berries with a tablespoon of sweetener and stir to coat. Set aside.

In a medium bowl, combine the almond flour, walnuts, remaining 2 tablespoons of sweetener, butter, vanilla extract, cinnamon, and salt. Stir with a fork until thoroughly combined. Scatter the nut mixture evenly over the berries and bake for 30 minutes or until lightly browned.

CALORIES 285 | PROTEIN 5 G (7%) | CARBS 12 G (16%) | FAT 25 G (77%)
SAT FAT 8.4 G | FIBER 5 G

3 cups mixed berries, fresh or frozen

3 tablespoons Swerve or another granulated zero-carb sweetener, divided

1½ cups almond flour

½ cup chopped walnuts

½ cup butter, softened

1 teaspoon vanilla extract

½ teaspoon ground cinnamon

Pinch of salt

RICOTTA-FILLED CREPES
with Blackberries

THESE SWEET CREPES make a beautiful presentation, but they're surprisingly easy to put together once you get the hang of it. If you're not a blackberry fan, use whatever type of berry you'd prefer.

MAKES 4 SERVINGS

1 cup ricotta

1 tablespoon lemon zest (optional)

4 ounces cream cheese

4 eggs

¼ cup Swerve or another granulated zero-carb sweetener

Pinch of salt

Dash of ground cinnamon

3 tablespoons butter

1 pint blackberries (about 2 cups)

In the work bowl of a food processor, whirl the ricotta and lemon zest (if using) until smooth and fluffy. Transfer the ricotta to a bowl and scrape out the work bowl. Add the cream cheese, eggs, sweetener, salt, and cinnamon to the work bowl and process until smooth.

In a 10-inch skillet, melt about 1 teaspoon of butter over medium-high heat. Working in batches, pour about 2 tablespoons of the egg mixture into the skillet and tilt it so that the batter evenly coats the bottom. Cook for 1 to 2 minutes until the top is set. Flip the crepe and cook for another 30 seconds until it begins to brown. Transfer to a plate and repeat with the remaining ingredients (you should have 8 crepes).

Spread about 2 tablespoons of the ricotta in the center of a crepe and roll it up, placing it seam-side down on a serving plate. Repeat with the remaining ingredients. Scatter the berries on top of the crepes and serve.

CALORIES 385 | PROTEIN 16 G (16%) | CARBS 10 G (10%) | FAT 32 G (74%)
SAT FAT 17.6 G | FIBER 4 G

PECAN-PUMPKIN FUDGE

WHILE IT TAKES A LITTLE TIME TO PUT TOGETHER, this nutty pumpkin fudge is a good reminder that berries and chocolate aren't the only means to a satisfying dessert when you're following a ketogenic weight loss plan. If you don't have much of a sweet tooth, you might want to omit the sweetener, as the coconut and pumpkin are naturally sweet.

MAKES 18 SERVINGS (2 PIECES EACH)

Preheat the oven to 350°F. Line a baking sheet with parchment paper. Line an 8- x 8-inch baking pan with aluminum foil so that it hangs over the sides, which will make the finished fudge easier to remove.

Scatter the pecans on the baking sheet. Bake for 5 to 8 minutes, stirring once or twice, until evenly toasted. Transfer the nuts to a plate and let cool. Set the parchment paper aside.

In the work bowl of a food processor, combine the coconut, sweetener, coconut oil, and a pinch of salt and process until the coconut is completely smooth and reaches a butter-like consistency. This may take up to 10 minutes and require stopping to scrape down the bowl several times.

In a small pot, cook the coconut mixture over medium low heat until the coconut is melted. Remove from the heat and add the pumpkin, cinnamon, and nutmeg. Stir until thoroughly combined.

Transfer the pumpkin mixture to the prepared baking pan and use the back of a spoon to spread it evenly. Scatter the toasted pecans on top. Lay the parchment paper on top and press evenly with your hands until the top is smooth. Refrigerate for 4 hours until firm. Lift the fudge from the pan, remove the foil, and cut into 36 pieces. Place in an airtight container and refrigerate up to a week. Let the fudge come to room temperature before serving.

CALORIES 225 | PROTEIN 3 G (5%) | CARBS 6 G (10%) | FAT 22 G (85%)
SAT FAT 15.5 G | FIBER 5 G

1 cup pecans, coarsely chopped

1 pound unsweetened shredded coconut

2 tablespoons Swerve or another granulated zero-carb sweetener

1 tablespoon coconut oil, melted

Pinch of salt

1 cup canned pumpkin puree

1 teaspoon ground cinnamon

¼ teaspoon ground nutmeg

DARK AND SALTY COCONUT ALMOND BARK

CLEARLY YOU DON'T NEED TO GIVE UP CANDY altogether when you're going low-carb. This quick little recipe is just the ticket when you crave a sweet treat.

MAKES 8 SERVING

½ cup almonds, coarsely chopped

½ cup unsweetened shredded coconut

¾ cup sugar-free chocolate chips

2 tablespoons butter

½ teaspoon almond extract

¼ teaspoon salt

Preheat the oven to 350°F. Line a baking sheet with parchment paper.

Scatter the almonds and coconut on the baking sheet. Bake for 5 to 8 minutes, stirring once or twice until evenly toasted. Transfer the nuts and coconut to a plate and let cool. Leave the parchment paper on the baking sheet.

Place the chocolate chips and butter in a microwavable bowl. Microwave on HIGH for 1 to 2 minutes until the chocolate melts. Add the almond extract and stir until thoroughly combined.

Pour the chocolate onto the parchment paper and spread evenly so the chocolate is about ¼-inch thick. Scatter the toasted nuts and coconut on top, pressing lightly so it adheres to the chocolate. Sprinkle with salt. Refrigerate until the chocolate is set. Use a knife or pizza cutter to break the candy into pieces before serving. Store in a cool, dark place.

CALORIES 220 | PROTEIN 2 G (4%) | CARBS 3 G (7%) | FAT 18 G (89%)
SAT FAT 10.7 G | FIBER 3 G

index